Prayer That Moves Mountains!

by Gordon Lindsay

Published by
Christ For The Nations, Inc.
P.O. Box 769000
Dallas, TX 75376-9000

Tenth Reprint 1998

All Scripture NKJV unless otherwise noted.

CONTENTS

CHAPTER I

Prayer That Moves Mountains

Jesus said, "Assuredly, I say to you, if you have faith and do not doubt, you will not only do what was done to the fig tree, but also if you say to this mountain, 'Be removed and be cast into the sea,' it will be done. And all things, whatever you ask in prayer, believing, you will receive" (Matt. 21:21,22).

Power to move mountains! That is what Jesus said you could have. His promise includes more — "all things." It sounds too good to be true, but it is true.

Perhaps at this moment you are weighted down with a heavy burden. It may be that you or a member of your family have a serious illness. Or maybe you are wrestling with financial problems. A solution to every problem is at your fingertips. God's power is waiting to set you free!

Do you have access to power that will move mountains? Yes! But you must learn the secret to releasing this power. Just wishing things will get better won't bring results. You may have found this out already. But the right kind of prayer — the kind Jesus spoke about when He said, "If you ask anything in My name, I will do it," (Jn. 14:14) — will bring the answer without fail.

Perhaps one of the most common ways people's faith is weakened is by assuming it is not God's will to answer their prayers.

While it is true that sometimes people ask for things not in His will, many things asked of God are in harmony with His revealed will. It is the will of God for the sick to be healed. It is the will of God that Christians live in good health. It is the will of God that believers have victory over oppression and fear. It is the will of God that His children's daily needs be supplied. It is the will of God that those in the body of Christ have the joy of the Lord in their hearts. It is the will of God that you prosper and be in health just as our soul prospers (III Jn. 2).

Let's get this straight. God doesn't want His people to be reconciled to defeat and failure. He wants them to have tangible results from praying — just as people did in Bible days. Prayer is an essential part of daily life. When you learn the secret of praying, miracles will become part of your life.

Consider God's mighty answers to prayer in the Bible. In his old age, Abraham desired a child of his wife, Sarah. God miraculously strengthened Sarah's womb so that she could bear him a son (Gen. 21:2).

Jacob, the grandson of Abraham, sought adventure, but later became a prince with God. Knowing his brother Esau was riding toward him with an army seeking vengeance, he wrestled with God during a night of prayer. Jacob prevailed with God, so God prevailed over Esau (Gen. 32,33).

Gideon hesitated to perform the task God had given him to do. Wanting to be absolutely sure he was in God's will, he asked God to make it clear. For a sign, on the first night he asked that the fleece would be wet and the ground dry. It was so. On the next night, he asked that the ground would be wet and the fleece dry. God answered his prayer. With the assurance that he was in God's will, Gideon won a victory that resulted in the liberation of his nation from a cruel oppressor (Judg. 6:36-40).

Samson achieved a great victory over the Philistines, but afterward was very thirsty. He called on the Lord God. Water came out of a hollow place in the jawbone Samson had used in battle (Judg. 15:18,19).

Solomon found himself king over the greatest empire on earth, but realized he was only a child in understanding. He prayed that God would give him the necessary wisdom to discharge his great responsibility. God made him the wisest man of his generation.

Jerusalem was invaded by a superior force of Assyrians who had been invariably successful in all their previous battles. Hezekiah's troops were no match for this great army. So Hezekiah prayed, and that night an angel of the Lord struck the invading host. By morning 185,000 men lay dead (II Ki. 19:15-35).

Shortly afterward, Hezekiah became deathly ill. In the natural, there was no hope of recovery. But Hezekiah turned his face to the wall and pled with God. As a result, 15 more years were added to his life (II Ki. 20:1-11).

Jabez was distressed by the wickedness of his day. He cried out to God, "Enlarge my territory, that Your hand would be with me, and that You would keep me from evil, that I may not cause pain!" (I Chron. 4:10). God granted him what he requested!

Jonah, the self-willed prophet, was thrown into the sea and swallowed by a big fish. After Jonah repented of his disobedience, God caused the fish to vomit him out on dry land and his life was spared (Jon. 2).

While Elijah was staying with the widow, her son grew ill and died. Elijah prayed and asked the Lord to restore life to the child. Never before had life returned to any person who had died. There was no precedent for raising the dead. Yet the prayer of Elijah caused the dead boy to revive (I Ki. 17:20-23).

Daniel prayed for the restoration of Jerusalem, which had been lying in ashes since the days of Nebuchadnezzar's invasion. The faithful prophet lived to see King Cyrus make a decree permitting all Jews who would, to return and rebuild their city (Dan. 9).

Habakkuk prayed for revival saying, "Revive Your work in the midst of the years! In the midst of the years make it known; in wrath remember mercy" (Hab. 3:2). His prayer was answered with perhaps the greatest and the last revival that occurred in the history of the kingdom of Judah (II Ki. 23:21-25).

Peter was cast into prison with orders for his execution. But the Church prayed without ceasing for his release, and an angel of the Lord visited the prison and led Peter to safety (Acts 12:3-11).

God has answered prayer for every conceivable need of His people, and under every imaginable circumstance. Whether it was deliverance from sickness, a miracle of supply, preservation from danger, divine guidance, saving one from dying of thirst, or for needed wisdom in ruling a kingdom — no matter what the need was — God supplied it in answer to believing prayer.

Jesus said, "Ask, and it will be given to you; seek, and you will find; knock, and it will be opened to you. For everyone who asks receives, and he who seeks finds, and to him who knocks it will be opened" (Matt. 7:7,8). What does this mean? It means there is an invisible power with us, able to work out every problem, anticipate every need, and supply whatever may be required — a power so great it can move mountains if need be. Does this sound too good to be true? As God is true, so is His promise. Your prayers can be answered too — if you will take time to learn the secret.

CHAPTER II

The Secret of the Presence of God

In Christ's first recorded sermon, He laid down some great principles that govern the successful operation of prayer. Jesus was interested only in prayer that brought the answer, and if need be, move mountains.

It was the habit of Jesus to always strike right at the heart of a matter. He knew what was essential. He didn't have to tell people to pray — that instinct was born in their hearts. The most ignorant heathen prayed. The prophets of Baal prayed. The hypocritical Pharisees prayed. Jesus was interested in showing believers the right way to pray, so they could have miracles in answer to their prayers.

THE SECRET CLOSET

Jesus started at the beginning. He showed that true prayer was communion with the Supreme Being — the Father God. Prayer was a solemn act and should be done the right way. He said that before praying one should seclude himself to be free from interruption. A person cannot successfully carry on human and divine communications at the same time. Jesus instructed that one should go into his room, shut the door and then pray to the Heavenly Father Who "sees in secret."

To emphasize His point, He mentioned the pharisees who prayed on the street corners to be seen of men. He cautioned His disciples not to be like them.

> And when you pray, you shall not be like the hypocrites. For they love to pray standing in the synagogues and on the corners of the streets, that they may be seen by men. Assuredly, I say to you, they have their reward. But you, when you pray, go into your room, and when you have shut your door, pray to your Father who is in the secret place; and your Father who sees in secret will reward you openly (Matt. 6:5,6).

Why must you get alone to pray? Because in prayer, you are entering into the presence of God. When you pray, you must be conscious of approaching your Creator, the One Who is worthy of absolute reverence and respect. The Old Testament writer wisely said:

> Do not be rash with your mouth, and let not your heart utter anything hastily before God. For God is in heaven, and you on earth; therefore let your words be few (Eccl. 5:2).

Most everyone knows that God is in heaven, *but the great secret of prayer is to realize and understand that He is also in the very room where you are*. It is the realization that God is actually present that makes prayer vital and powerful. When you realize that God is in the very room where you are, you will not be careless in your conversation with Him. As Jesus said, "But when you pray, do not use vain repetitions as the heathen do. For they think that they will be heard for their many words" (Matt. 6:7).

God is in heaven, but He is also on earth. When David was being chased by Saul, he was tempted to believe God was so far off He might not be able to save him in time (I Sam. 27:1). David learned that wherever he was, God was present also. He acknowledged this, although in Psalm 139:6-10 he admitted he did not fully understand it:

Such knowledge is too wonderful for me; it is high, I cannot attain it. Where can I go from Your Spirit? Or where can I flee from Your presence? If I ascend into heaven, You are there; if I make my bed in hell, behold, You are there. If I take the wings of the morning, and dwell in the uttermost parts of the sea, even there Your hand shall lead me, and Your right hand shall hold me.

GOD IS EVERYWHERE — HE DOESN'T COME AND HE DOESN'T GO

God is everywhere. He doesn't come and He doesn't go. He is the great I AM! Jesus showed that worshiping God is not to be confined to a certain place or a certain time. The woman of Samaria wanted to know which was the proper place to worship — Jerusalem or a mountain nearby. This question was the subject of bitter controversy in that day and it occurred to the woman that this was a golden opportunity to get a prophet's answer. Jesus answered her question in a way she hardly expected. He said,

Woman, believe Me, the hour is coming when you will neither on this mountain, nor in Jerusalem, worship the Father ... But the hour is coming, and now is, when the true worshipers will worship the Father in spirit and truth; for the Father is seeking such to worship Him (Jn. 4:21,23).

WE MUST RECOGNIZE THE PRESENCE OF GOD

Recognizing the presence of God makes it easy to pray and have faith. Though God is not visibly present, He is present just the same. Recognizing this actual presence of God, prayer no longer is a chore, but a supreme delight. The Lord made it clear that Christ's presence is always with His people.

Jesus answered and said to him, "If anyone loves Me, he will keep My word; and My Father will love him, and We will come to him and make Our home with him" (Jn. 14:23).

Failure to recognize the presence of the Lord in daily life makes it difficult to recognize His presence as one prays. The recognition of the presence of God is the first great secret of prayer.

THOSE WHO WERE MIGHTY IN PRAYER RECOGNIZED GOD'S PRESENCE

Those who had outstanding power in prayer in Bible days were the ones who learned the secret of the presence of the Lord. Abraham the patriarch met the Lord in the company of angels at his tent door (Gen. 18:1). During that wonderful hour of fellowship, Abraham received boldness to intercede for the city of Sodom. Although he was unable to stop judgment on the city brought on by their grievous wickedness, his nephew Lot and his wife and daughters were warned and given the opportunity to escape.

Moses, the mighty intercessor, stood in the gap between Israel and judgment. He prayed:

> Oh, these people have sinned a great sin, and have made for themselves a god of gold! Yet now, if You will forgive their sin — but if not, I pray, blot me out of Your book which You have written (Ex. 32:31,32).

There had been a time when Moses tried to liberate the children of Israel by natural means. But his efforts failed. Years later at the burning bush, he met the One Who revealed Himself as the I AM THAT I AM. From that day on, God was an ever-present reality to Moses. No longer a failure, Moses became the great intercessor of the Old Testament. When the children of Israel sinned, the Lord refused to continue with them on their journey to Canaan. Moses would have none of it. He said, "If Your Presence does not go with us, do not bring us up from here" (Ex. 33:15). And he persuaded the Lord to grant his request. God reassured him, saying:

> I will also do this thing that you have spoken; for you have found grace in My sight, and I know you by name (Ex. 33:17).

Daniel was another mighty man of prayer. In a vision he saw God ascend His very throne. He watched as the "Ancient of Days" sat down in judgment while millions ministered to Him. He saw "One like the Son of Man, coming with the clouds of heaven! He came to the Ancient of Days, and they brought Him near before Him" (Dan. 7:13). These vivid experiences made the presence of the Lord more real to Daniel than the presence of the king, princes, or even the lions in the den. Now that the Holy Spirit has come, God's presence is with believers in a unique manner.

The day came when Jesus was to leave His disciples. How they longed for Him to stay with them! But Jesus explained why He must leave: "If I do not go away, the Helper will not come to you" (Jn. 16:7). Through the Holy Spirit Jesus could be present, not with just a few, but with all believers everywhere. He could then fulfill His promise that "where two or three are gathered together in My name, I am there in the midst of them" (Matt. 18:20).

What is the first secret of prayer? What is the secret to moving mountains by the prayer of faith? The first requirement is to recognize the presence of Him who created mountains. Recognize that Christ is with you every moment. Then it will be easy to recognize the presence of Christ when you pray. Start recognizing and practicing the presence of Christ in your life.

CHAPTER III

The Secret of Praise

In this manner, therefore, pray: *Our Father in heaven, hallowed be Your name.* Your kingdom come. Your will be done on earth as it is in heaven. Give us this day our daily bread. And forgive us our debts, As we forgive our debtors. And do not lead us into temptation, but deliver us from the evil one. *For Yours is the kingdom and the power and the glory forever.* Amen (Matt. 6:9-13).

You want to learn the secret of prayer that will move mountains — prayer that will change things; that will tap the infinite resources of Almighty God; that will make the invisible become visible; that will release the power of heaven for the benefit of humanity? Well, you can learn the secret, but you must be willing to follow God's rules.

THE DISCIPLES SAID, "LORD, TEACH US TO PRAY"

In Luke's account of the Lord's prayer (read Luke 11:1-4), the disciples said to Jesus, "Lord, teach us to pray." There was a reason they asked this question. The disciples had watched Jesus as He healed the sick. They had seen Him cleanse the leper with the touch of His hand. They had witnessed His healing power to the blind and the deaf. They had observed that even the elements responded to His command. At His word the winds were stilled — as He spoke, the waves of the angry sea were calmed. How was He able to do these things? What was the secret to such mighty power?

At first it all seemed a mystery, but gradually the disciples learned the secret. Jesus had this power because He knew how to pray! Soon they wanted to learn how to pray, too. One day they asked Jesus if He would teach them.

The Lord did not hesitate to grant their request. He was not One to keep His secrets to Himself. People have often tried to monopolize power — but not Christ. He came into the world to teach others to do what He did. He was willing that His disciples should learn to do even *greater* works (Jn. 14:12).

Yes, He would teach them to pray. And He began by telling them to pray in this manner: "Our Father in heaven, hallowed be Your name" (Matt. 6:9). He concluded His model prayer with these words: "For Yours is the kingdom and the power and the glory forever. Amen" (Matt. 6:13). In these sentences, Christ revealed a second great secret of prayer: Prayer that reaches God, begins and ends with worship!

PRAYER BEGINS WITH WORSHIP

God is great and good. All that you are or will be is entirely due to Him, the Giver of "every good gift and perfect gift" (Jas. 1:17). Therefore, as a creature to his Creator, you and I owe God our sincere worship and praise. Worship is the first element in prayer.

This is where some make their mistake. They think of prayer as a means to receive help in an emergency. True, that is one purpose of prayer, but certainly not the only purpose. If necessary, God will move mountains or stop the sun and moon in their courses to help one of His children. But He also wants something from our prayer. What could God possibly want? He Who is eternal, the All-Sufficient One — what could a mere human have to offer to Him Who rules the universe?

There is one thing God seeks and longs for — worship. Since the creature owes everything to the Creator, it is right and proper they should worship Him. We should praise the Lord every day of our lives. As the last verse in the Book of Psalms declares, "Let everything that has breath praise the LORD. Praise the LORD!" (Psa. 150:6).

In the first chapter, we mentioned the woman at Jacob's well. She asked where was the best place to worship. Christ gave her one of His greatest revelations. He said, "But the hour is coming, and now is, when the true worshipers will worship the Father in spirit and truth; for the *Father is seeking such to worship Him*" (Jn. 4:23). God seeks one thing from the human race — one thing they can give — worship in spirit and in truth.

When Jesus was on earth, He revealed the fact that the religious people of that day had made prayer into a form. One sect claimed men should worship God only in Jerusalem. Another said the proper place to worship was on Mount Gerizim in Samaria. But Jesus proclaimed that neither Jerusalem nor some mountain were necessarily where people should pray. God is Spirit; He is everywhere. Therefore, He wants everyone to worship Him wherever they are.

Satan competes with God for the worship of men. When the devil tempted Christ, he promised Him the kingdoms and glory of this world, if only He would fall down and worship him (Matt. 4:9). Jesus rejected Satan's offer and told him worship was reserved for God alone.

Notice how Christ gave thanksgiving and praise to God while praying. His first recorded prayer was, "I thank You, Father, Lord of heaven and earth, because You have hidden these things from the wise and prudent and have revealed them to babes" (Matt. 11:25). Before Christ raised Lazarus from the tomb, He thanked God for hearing Him (Jn. 11:41). As Jesus made His triumphal entry into Jerusalem, He was urged to rebuke the little children as they praised the Lord. Instead He said, "Yes. Have you never read, 'Out of the mouth of babes and nursing infants You have perfected praise?'" (Matt. 21:16).

PRAISE BRINGS THE BAPTISM OF THE HOLY GHOST

In Luke's version of the Lord's prayer, Jesus concludes by saying, "If you then, being evil, know how to give good gifts to your children, how much more will your heavenly Father give the Holy Spirit to those who ask Him!" (Lk. 11:13). The following is the writer's testimony on receiving the Holy Spirit:

After conversion, I read the above promise. My heart was hungry for the baptism of the Holy Spirit. I wanted that experience more than anything else in the world. Night after night, I told God I would do anything within my power if He would grant me that blessing.

But I first had to learn the secret of praise. I prayed, but I didn't know how to praise the Lord. Fortunately, others showed me that I should quit begging and begin to praise God for the answer. Since I had asked the Lord for the blessing, I should now start thanking Him for it. I did not know very much about praying, but did what they told me. Lifting my hands toward heaven, I thanked God for His promise that He would grant me the baptism of the Holy Spirit. I shall never forget what happened! The apostle Peter was right when he said we have not followed cunningly devised fables (II Pet. 1:16). The baptism of the Holy Ghost is not a figment of our imagination. It is a river of living water; a dynamic pouring out of divine power. It is an intense reality.

The Holy Ghost came upon me in surges of power that flowed down through my whole being. Waves of heavenly glory, like electricity but infinitely pleasant, rolled over me until they engulfed my whole being. Conversion had changed my life, but now the baptism of the Holy Ghost transformed it.

The great secret I learned was that praise brings the blessing. I have seen people beg for the Holy Ghost and go away empty-handed; others came praising God, and received in a moment of time. Once you learn the secret of praise, it is not difficult to receive from God.

It was when the "trumpeters and singers were as one, to make one sound to be heard in praising and thanking the LORD," (II Chron 5:13) that Solomon's temple was filled with the glory of God.

When the disciples were praising and blessing God (Lk. 24:52,53), the Holy Ghost came and "filled the whole house where they were sitting" (Acts 2:2).

During a time of great despondency among the early settlers of America, it was proposed that a fast be called. But one farmer spoke out against always provoking heaven with complaints. He suggested instead they have a day of thanksgiving, pointing out they had much to be thankful for. His suggestion was accepted and a day of thanksgiving was appointed. The custom has continued in America ever since.

God is more than the Creator, He is the Father of all mankind. We are the "offspring of God" (Acts 17:29), and made in His image and likeness (Gen. 1:26). Praise should be as natural to the creature as breathing. Unfortunately, the image of God has been marred by sin. Fallen man feels a revulsion to worshiping His Creator. Because of sin, man has cut himself off from God and is out of relationship with Him.

The great miracle is that God made a way for us to return to Him. "But God, who is rich in mercy, because of His great love with which He loved us, even when we were dead in trespasses, made us alive together with Christ" (Eph. 2:4,5). Through Christ, communion with the Father is restored!

There is only one prayer the sinner can pray and be heard by God: "God be merciful to me a sinner!" (Lk. 18:13). Once forgiven, a man or woman is renewed by the Spirit of God and communion is restored. Then we are able to praise and worship God the Creator.

PRAISE IS THE KEY TO ENTERING GOD'S PRESENCE

"Enter into His gates with thanksgiving, And into His courts with praise. Be thankful to Him, and bless His name. For the LORD is good; His mercy is everlasting, And His truth endures to all generations" (Psa. 100:4,5). If you want something from God, thank Him for what He has already done. People are often quick to ask God for help, but slow to thank Him for the answer He so graciously gives. Ten lepers came to Jesus to be healed, but only one returned afterwards to give God thanks (Lk. 17:17,18). Those who need deliverance should thank God for what He has already done. They are then likely to receive more.

Asking should always be mingled with praise and thanksgiving. "Be anxious for nothing, but in everything by prayer and supplication, with thanksgiving, let your requests be made known to God" (Phil. 4:6).

Jesus said that those who believe shall "say to this mountain, 'Be removed and be cast into the sea,' it will be done" (Matt. 21:21). But before the Lord spoke these words He also said, "Yes. Have you never read, 'Out of the mouth of babes and nursing infants You have perfected praise?'" (Matt. 21:16). Those who desire to move mountains should learn to praise.

The secret of praise and thanksgiving is important in the art of prayer. Enter into God's presence with praise. Bring your requests to God with thanksgiving. Praise Him for what He has already done. The powers of heaven and earth, the power to move mountains, is at the bidding of those who have learned the secret of praise. Start the habit today of giving Him the sacrifice of praise continually (Heb. 13:15).

CHAPTER IV

The Secret of World Vision

Pray ... Your kingdom come. Your will be done on earth as it is in heaven (Matt. 6:9,10).

Now it shall come to pass in the latter days that the mountain of the Lord's house shall be established on the top of the mountains, and shall be exalted above the hills; and all nations shall flow to it. ... He shall judge between the nations, and shall rebuke many people; they shall beat their swords into plowshares, and their spears into pruning hooks; nation shall not lift up sword against nation, neither shall they learn war anymore (Isa. 2:2,4).

Jesus' statement that prayer has power to move mountains often puzzles people. They think the word "mountains" must be figurative. Surely the Lord did not mean that a real mountain could be moved by prayer.

It is true that "mountain" is often used figuratively in Scripture but this does not lessen the force of Christ's promise. The word "mountain" is often symbolic of a kingdom. Christ's kingdom is spoken of in Daniel 2:35 as a "great mountain" that "filled the whole earth."

In Isaiah 2:2, Isaiah refers to the "mountain of the Lord's house," to the kingdom of God that is to be established upon the earth. It is a kingdom that will result in universal peace, with the nations beating "their swords into plowshares and their spears into pruninghooks" (Isa. 2:4).

How is this great "mountain of the Lord's house" — the kingdom of God — to be established on earth? It will come as the result of the prayers of God's people! Jesus indicated this in the prayer He taught His disciples when He said, "Pray ... Your kingdom come. Your will be done on earth as it is in heaven" (Matt. 6:9,10).

Christ would not ask His people to pray for something that would come to pass anyway. He never told believers to pray for the sun to rise, because it will rise regardless. But He did tell His Church to pray for His kingdom to come — a kingdom that would supercede the kingdoms of this world (Rev. 11:15;16:20).

THE KINGDOM MUST FIRST COME INTO HEARTS OF MEN

Will the kingdom drop out of heaven as a result of prayer? No, Jesus made it plain that it would not come that way. He said, "The kingdom of God does not come with observation; nor will they say, 'See here!' or 'See there!' For indeed, the kingdom of God is within you" (Lk. 17:20,21). Christ must rule *in* the hearts of men before He will reign *over* them. The supreme work of the followers of Christ is to preach the kingdom of God, that it might enter into the hearts of men. This great task was begun by the apostles, but is still unfinished today. Christ expressly stated that, "This gospel of the kingdom will be preached in all the world as a witness to all the nations, and then the end will come" (Matt. 24:14).

From His great position on the throne, God looks over the earth and sees all the sorrow and woe caused by sin and the broken law. He yearns for the redemption of the whole earth. He so loved the world that He gave His only begotten Son. He is waiting for vast populations who have never heard the name of Jesus to be evangelized. What is the Church doing about this?

The truth is the prayers of the Church are weak because of its narrow vision. A vast number of Christians pray only for their personal interests. How many churches are really interested in world evangelization? How many have an interest in God's work outside of their own denomination? We must broaden our vision to wider horizons. World evangelization can only be brought about by the *united effort of the whole body of Christ*. Only then will the world believe that Christ is the Son of God.

> That they all may be one, as You, Father, are in Me, and
> I in You; that they also may be one in Us, *that the world*
> *may believe that You sent Me* (Jn. 17:21).

Now is the time for the Church to pray as Jesus taught, "Your kingdom come. Your will be done on earth as it is in heaven" (Matt. 6:10). Let the Church pray for its members to become one so the world may believe Jesus Christ is indeed sent of the Father. Those who will pray this unselfish prayer may also pray, "Give us this day our daily bread" (Matt. 6:11), and they will not wait long for the answer.

The sin of selfishness has been from the beginning. "You ask and do not receive, because you ask amiss, that you may spend it on your pleasures" (Jas. 4:3). Prayer is not to be a convenient device for gratifying ambitious or selfish desires. God wants Christians to pray for their own needs, but He also wants them to pray for the coming of the kingdom. As the Church shares God's burden of a lost world, He will share their burden.

A PERSONAL VISION OF WORLD REVIVAL

Shortly after my conversion, God gave me a vision of world revival. The call of the Gospel absorbed my whole being to the extent that all other ambitions in life faded. I found that I would rather preach the Gospel than do anything else in the world.

Much of our evangelistic work was done during the depression years. Those were the days when one could prove whether or not he had a call from God. Often an evangelist might find that his love offering at the end of the week amounted to $3-5. But however small the financial remuneration, my wife and I can truthfully say that never did we have the slightest temptation to leave the ministry.

But in one area we were greatly dissatisfied. The results were not in proportion to the overwhelming need. The Church was winning the lost one by one, but this was not a drop in the bucket as far as world evangelization was concerned. It was plain from the Scriptures that God intended the Gospel of the kingdom be preached as a witness unto all nations. He said, "Preach the gospel to every creature" (Mk. 16:15). But at the rate it was going, we could see the job would never be accomplished.

During those days God showed us — as well as many others — that a revival was coming that would reach the masses. How we prayed and looked forward to it. A revival that would reach the whole world! One that would reach audiences of tens of thousands!

Then God sent the revival! By a series of strange providences, we were brought into the center of it. It was the privilege of my wife and me to share in the organization of the first meeting of those involved in this visitation. As time went on, it was our joy to see many of our colleagues participating in great campaigns in foreign lands — reaching tens, even hundreds of thousands. Whole nations were being stirred. Where missionaries had labored arduously for years with meager results, mighty visitations came. The revival proved to be of a scope never before known in history.

Thank God for those to whom He has given a world vision. In praying "Your kingdom come. Your will be done on earth as it is in heaven" (Matt. 6:10), they are receiving a rich reward.

This is but a token of what is to come. Before the Church lies a time of still greater accomplishments. It is time to pray for revival more far-reaching than any that has been known before. May God give the body of Christ a vision of world revival — a revival that goes beyond organizations or denominations, one that will take in the whole Church. Those who pray "Your kingdom come," will find their personal needs will be taken care of.

THE VITAL NEED OF THE CHURCH IS WORLD VISION

The vital need of the Church at the present time is a world vision. The greatest hindrance to the Church receiving that vision is its preoccupation with its own programs. God's people must be willing to work together, regardless of denominations. It has become difficult to reach sinners in a local church, but they can still be reached through believers' unified efforts. If Christians will back such efforts, even though they may not gain a single member for their own body, they will witness a startling advance in the evangelization of their community. In the end every church will receive its share of the blessing.

Before a believer can learn the secret of moving mountains by prayer, he must accept a world vision. He must pray for the harvest of the world. He must pray for the evangelization of a billion souls without Christ. He must pray that God's kingdom will come and His will be done on earth. He who prays this prayer unselfishly will see mountains moved — and his own needs will be met.

CHAPTER V

The Secret of Praying in the Will of God

Your will be done on earth as it is in heaven (Matt. 6:10).

And though I have all faith, so that I could remove mountains, but have not love (divine love), I am nothing (I Cor. 13:2).

God has promised you power to move mountains, but you must be sure to move the ones *He* wants moved. God never puts His power on display for no reason, nor does He give special demonstrations for entertainment. The moving of a mountain is of no benefit unless it accomplishes a purpose in the will of God — and unless the act is motivated by a love for humanity. As Paul said, faith to move mountains is meaningless without love.

The important factor is the will of God. It is necessary that when you pray, "Your will be done on earth as it is in heaven," you seek the will of God to be done in your life. As I John 5:14 says, "Now this is the confidence that we have in Him, that if we ask anything according to His will, He hears us."

MANKIND IS GOD'S MASTERPIECE

Mankind is the crowning glory of God's creation. Adam and Eve were made in the image and likeness of God and given dominion over the earth (Gen. 1:26). Their home was in the Garden of Eden, and in this paradise there was no sin, sickness, pain, suffering or death. Before they chose to disobey God, all things moved in the orbit of God's perfect will.

In the Garden an evil choice was made, and mankind moved out of the will of God. God countermoved to save the human race by sending Christ into the world. Those who are redeemed have all that Adam and Eve originally possessed — and more. Through Christ every good thing is available for the asking. As Jesus said:

> Ask, and it will be given to you; seek, and you will find; knock, and it will be opened to you. For everyone who asks receives, and he who seeks finds, and to him who knocks it will be opened (Lk. 11:9,10).

Why is it then, that so many of God's children seem unable to appropriate the promise? Why are their prayers not answered? Why do so few miracles happen in their lives? Why is it that no mountains are moved? Could it be that there is something missing, something lacking in their lives that deprives them of the benefit of the promise?

THE MYSTERY OF UNANSWERED PRAYER

There is a key to unfolding the mystery of unanswered prayer. God has a pattern and a purpose for every person born into this world. The greatest moment in a Christian's experience is discovering that purpose for existence.

When a believer is operating in the will of God for his life, the powers of heaven and earth work for his good. "All things work together for good to those who love God, to those who are the called according to His purpose" (Rom. 8:28).

When you become absolutely committed to the will of God, you will discover that the most vexing problems of life have a mysterious way of working themselves out. How does this happen? The God Who made the planets, the sun, the moon and the stars, and Who causes them to follow in their appointed paths by His irresistible will, causes all things in our lives to follow also in the proper orbit.

HOW GOD SHOWED US HIS WILL IN BUILDING THE VOICE OF HEALING PLANT

The importance of God's will in accomplishing anything worthwhile became very clear in our work with The Voice of Healing. In 1951, we contemplated building offices in Dallas. At that time we had no money to pay for the project. We knew this move must be absolutely in God's divine will if it were to succeed. We prayed daily. At one point we were ready to move, but God stopped us. Those who wait on the Lord cannot be in a hurry. We continued to pray. Finally the hour came when God said, "Now is the time. Rise and build." We were certain that we were moving in the will of God.

But every step needed to be carefully prayed through. First, we had to choose a building site. We almost made a deal on one lot. An unexpected legal technicality hindered us. Later we found out it would not have been adequate for our future growth. We did not fully realize what God had in store for us. But God kept us from making a mistake. In the meantime, we had a chance to locate a piece of property that would meet our requirements. The city planning commission had intended on zoning the area for residences, but through a clerk's error we were given permission to build. Though the mistake was discovered, the commission decided to let us go ahead. We felt that the location was ideal and that God gave it to us.

Now came the critical moment. If God was in this move, He must supply the $20,000 we needed in a short time. Did God meet us? Yes, He did! The miracle took place, and in a few months we had a fine building erected. But it was only a small part of what we were going to need in the next few years.

Soon we needed to expand the growing ministries of The Voice of Healing. From where would the needed money come? God gave us the answer in an unexpected way. He blessed my ministry of writing, not only enabling me to support my family, but to continue our program of expansion. In addition, we received some liberal gifts which permitted us to move forward rapidly. Then we built

additional offices for a missions department. We erected a publica-
tion building and installed printing equipment for our literature
crusade. So in a few short years, we had a large well-equipped
establishment.

We have learned that when each step is prayed through and is
clearly in the will of God, the miracle that is needed will take place.

THE PILLAR OF CLOUD

God's plan for guiding His redeemed people is beautifully
illustrated in the story of how God led the children of Israel. They
knew they were to make the journey into the Promised Land. God
did not leave them to their own resources and wisdom — even in
making that short journey. They were led by the presence of the Lord
Who dwelt in the cloud of the Tabernacle. When the cloud moved
forward they went, and when it stopped, they stopped.

> When the cloud was taken up from above the tabernacle,
> the children of Israel went onward in all their journeys.
> But if the cloud was not taken up, then they did not
> journey till the day that it was taken up. For the cloud of
> the LORD was above the tabernacle by day, and fire was
> over it by night, in the sight of all the house of Israel,
> throughout all their journeys (Ex. 40:36-38).

It is solemn to note the generation of Israelites who refused to
follow the cloud, was never permitted to enter the Promised Land.
When they said, "Let us select a leader and return to Egypt" (Num.
14:4), they were rebelling against divine guidance and God left them
to die in the wilderness.

TO HAVE MIRACLES ONE'S LIFE MUST BE COMMITTED TO THE WILL OF GOD

Some want this or that person to pray for them, confessing that
God does not answer their prayers and their problems only become
greater. What is wrong? Why are these people so beaten? Could it
be that their life is out of the revealed will of God? That is usually

the reason for their consistent failure. Jesus said to pray, "Your will be done on earth as it is in heaven." To pray that prayer means, "Lord, let your will be done in my life." For the will of God can only be done in earth as it is done in our lives.

In the Garden of Gethsemane, Christ set the example of absolute committal to the will of God. There He came to grips with the powers of darkness. Yet even while His soul was tortured in the terrible struggle, He was able to pray, "O My Father, if it is possible, let this cup pass from Me; nevertheless, not as I will, but as You will" (Matt. 26:39). Christ resigned Himself to the will of God, though it meant drinking His cup to the bitter dregs.

If you are going to see mountains moved as Christ did, then you must pray like He did, "Not as I will, but as You will." If you are going to receive answers to prayer as He did, then you must commit yourself to the will of God. This means death to the self-life. But after death, resurrection life comes as compensation — and with it joy and peace in the Holy Ghost. Though Christ endured suffering in the closing hours of His earthly life, God also gave Him such joy that He could say, "These things I have spoken to you, that My joy may remain in you, and that your joy may be full" (Jn. 15:11).

Another important secret of prayer is to pray like Christ did, "Not my will but thine be done." Every step must be committed to God. It is important to seek God's will and His blessing, rather than asking Him to bless *our* plans. God will only grant the power to move mountains if it will accomplish His purposes. "If you abide in Me, and My words abide in you, you will ask what you desire, and it shall be done for you" (Jn. 15:7).

CHAPTER VI

The Secret of Knowing What to Pray For

Your will be done on earth as it is in heaven (Lk. 11:2).

It is important to know what *is* and what *is not* the will of God. Obviously, some prayers are not answered because they are clearly out of the revealed will of God. However, more people fail to receive because of lack of faith than from asking for something out of God's will. The fact is, many people avoid facing failure by assuming it was not God's will to give them what they asked — perhaps because of some mysterious divine purpose.

This is often the case with those who fail to receive healing. They claim God did not heal them because it was not His will. This, of course, is a serious error. It is denying the revealed will of God which says, "Who forgives all your iniquities, Who heals all your diseases" (Psa. 103:3). Since forgiveness and healing are mentioned in the same verse, denying the promise of healing is tantamount to denying God's willingness to forgive.

Nonetheless, there are petitions that go up to God that are obviously out of His will. Successful prayer means that we pray according to His will. God will move a mountain if need be, but it must have a purpose in God's divine will. In some instances, a prayer may be of a nature that it cannot be answered. During the American Civil War, soldiers on both sides gathered in prayer meetings and earnestly sought God to make their side win. Obviously, both sides could not win.

There are many things to pray for, where God's will is not open to question. At other times we must pray like Christ when He said, "Not my will but thine be done." One thing is certain, any revelation from God will never be contrary to what He has already revealed concerning His will in His Word.

There are prayers recorded in the Scriptures which were out of God's will and were not answered:

1. *Elijah's prayer that he might die* (I Ki. 19:4). God did not answer this prayer because He had a far different plan for Elijah. He was to be translated into heaven so that he would not see death. From our vantage point, we can see how foolish Elijah was to ask for death in an hour of discouragement, when such a great experience was ahead of him. Many since Elijah's day have prayed the same prayer. The believer should ask God to give strength and encouragement for each day, and leave his or her time of earthly departure to God.

2. *Balak's desire for Israel to be cursed* (Num. 22). Balak was terrified of the children of Israel and wanted them to be cursed so he could defeat them in battle. He said to the prophet Balaam, "Therefore please come at once, curse this people for me, for they are too mighty for me. Perhaps I shall be able to defeat them and drive them out of the land, for I know that he whom you bless is blessed, and he whom you curse is cursed" (Num. 22:6). The prophet Balaam was not committed to the revealed will of God. Even though the Lord told Balaam that Israel was not to be cursed, he still dallied with the king of Moab. Because there was a house full of silver as a reward, he tried to get further revelation from God about a matter that was already fully revealed.

3. *Jeremiah's prayer for blessing on people who rejected the will of God* (Jer. 14:1-16). Some people picture God as being ready to answer anybody's prayers whether or not they have any

intention of serving Him. No doubt, on occasion God has overlooked a sinner's ignorance and answered his prayer. But God will not normally answer prayer for those who rebel against His will and live a life of sin. In Jeremiah's day, the Israelites had forsaken the Lord and were in apostasy. Their prophets falsely prophesied peace and healing, but famine came instead (Jer. 14:19). A serious drought was upon the land and Jeremiah was praying that it would be broken. But God told Jeremiah, "Do not pray for this people, for their good. When they fast, I will not hear their cry; and when they offer burnt offering and grain offering, I will not accept them. But I will consume them by the sword, by the famine, and by the pestilence" (Jer. 14:11,12). When a nation has turned from God to idols, there is no use in praying for relief from judgment. The only way of escape is through repentance. An individual or a nation can sin to the extent that judgment is sure to come. "There is sin leading to death. I do not say that he should pray about that" (I Jn. 5:16).

4. *For destruction of enemies* (Lk. 9:55,56). When mercy is past, only judgment remains. But God always extends mercy before judgment. We live in a dispensation of God's mercy. Sometimes people are ready to execute judgment before God is. This happened to James and John. They had been treated unkindly and been turned away at a certain village in Samaria. James and John — true to their name — "Sons of Thunder," asked Jesus if they could destroy the village by calling fire from heaven. They said, "Lord, do You want us to command fire to come down from heaven and consume them, just as Elijah did?" (Lk. 9:54). They did not yet perceive that with the coming of Christ a new age of grace had dawned. They were to be motivated differently than those who lived under the law in the Old Testament days. Jesus rebuked the over-zealous disciples saying, "You do not know what manner of spirit you are of. For the Son of Man did not come to destroy men's lives but to save them" (Lk. 9:55,56).

5. *Covetous prayers.* Many prayers are motivated by covetousness. God has promised a hundred-fold return in this life, and in the

world to come, eternal life. But those who look upon prayer as merely a means of obtaining material benefits may well find their prayers unanswered. James says, "You ask and do not receive, because you ask amiss, that you may spend it on your pleasures" (Jas. 4:3).

One day a man approached Jesus requesting He use His position to persuade his brother to divide the inheritance with him. "Teacher, tell my brother to divide the inheritance with me" (Lk. 12:13). The Lord answered with a sharp rebuke, warning him and the others present with the story of the rich fool. This man's heart was centered on all the crops and goods gathered in his barns and said, "Soul ... take your ease; eat, drink, and be merry" (Lk. 12:19). But that very night God took an account and said to him, "You fool! This night your soul will be required of you" (Lk. 12:20). God does not bless a prayer that is motivated by a covetous spirit.

6. *Prayer for signs.* The Pharisees came to Jesus and asked Him to perform a sign for them. He refused their request and told them no sign would be given them except the sign of Jonah the prophet. There are people today who say they will believe if a certain person is healed, or if a certain miracle is performed. Herod was one who wanted to see Jesus because "he hoped to see some miracle done by Him" (Lk. 23:8). Jesus would not even talk to him, let alone perform a miracle. There are no miracles for the haughty — only for the humble of heart.

7. *Ambitious prayers.* James and John were ambitious and desired to be great, so they said to Jesus, "Teacher, we want You to do for us whatever we ask" (Mk. 10:35). They then explained that one of them wanted to sit on Jesus' right hand and the other on His left when He came into His glory. Their ambitious request produced envy and indignation among the other disciples. But Jesus showed there was no place for rivalry in the kingdom of God. He discouraged prayers motivated by ambition. "For whoever exalts himself will be abased, and he who humbles himself will be exalted" (Lk. 14:11).

WHAT TO PRAY FOR

Just as it is necessary to know what not to pray for, so it is important to know what to pray for. The Lord's prayer mentions several things for which believers should pray: For the kingdom of God to come on earth; supply of daily needs; forgiveness of sins; and deliverance from evil. Scripture mentions a number of other prayers that believers should pray:

1. *Pray to receive the Holy Spirit.* When Jesus was teaching His disciples how to pray, He said to them, "For everyone who asks receives, and he who seeks finds, and to him who knocks it will be opened" (Lk. 11:10). "If you then, being evil, know how to give good gifts to your children, how much more will your heavenly Father give the Holy Spirit to those who ask Him!" (Lk. 11:13).

   Why did Jesus say the Holy Spirit is the most important thing to ask for? Because the believer needs the Holy Spirit more than anything else. Without the Holy Spirit, he cannot pray effectively, he cannot defeat the devil, he cannot overcome self. "God be merciful to me a sinner," should be the first prayer of the sinner, and "God fill me with the Holy Spirit" should be the first prayer of the believer.

2. *Pray for those who spitefully use you* (Matt. 5:44). It is human to dislike an enemy. It is divine to pray for him. Jesus' command to pray for our enemies distinguishes Christianity from all other religions. Only the grace of God gives a man power to pray for someone who has injured him. But Jesus did that on the cross when He prayed, "Father, forgive them, for they do not know what they do" (Lk. 23:34). It is both remarkable and significant that Jesus' first teaching on prayer was about praying for our enemies.

3. *Pray that the Lord of the harvest will send laborers into His harvest.* The world will not be evangelized without believers doing their part. It is the Church's solemn obligation to pray for

God to raise up men who will carry this great message of deliverance to the ends of the earth. "Pray the Lord of the harvest to send out laborers into His harvest" (Lk. 10:2).

4. *Pray for the brethren.* Jesus said to Peter, "But I have prayed for you, that your faith should not fail; and when you have returned to Me, strengthen your brethren" (Lk. 22:32).

5. *Pray for protection and safety of God's ministers.* When Peter was in prison — expecting to be executed in the morning — the Church was praying for his deliverance. As a result, an angel came and opened the doors of the prison and led him to safety.

6. *Pray for those in authority.* Pray "for kings and all who are in authority, that we may lead a quiet and peaceable life in all godliness and reverence" (I Tim. 2:2).

7. *Pray that you will be counted worthy to stand before Christ at His coming.* "Watch therefore, and pray always that you may be counted worthy to escape all these things that will come to pass, and to stand before the Son of Man" (Lk. 21:36).

8. *Pray for the unity of all believers that the world may believe.* "That they all may be one, as You, Father, are in Me, and I in You; that they also may be one in Us, that the world may believe that You sent Me (Jn. 17:21).

9. *Pray for sick to be healed.* "Pray for one another, that you may be healed" (Jas. 5:16). There are some things we will know to be God's will only after we have earnestly prayed about the matter. But it is not honoring God to seek His will about something He has already declared as His will. For example, God said, "Go into all the world and preach the gospel to every creature. ... And these signs will follow those who believe: In My name they will cast out demons; ... they will lay hands on the sick, and they will recover" (Mk. 16:15,17,18). We are not to ask God if this is the way to evangelize the heathen. We are to do it!

TRIP TO MEXICO PROVES
GOD'S WILL IN EVANGELISM

In 1949, Freda and I decided to take a trip to Mexico. We were certain that the proper method to reach people in other lands was to pray for the sick, but we wanted to prove its practicality. With some reluctance, a Mexican pastor gave us permission to preach in his church. A rather unenthusiastic crowd was present at the first service. As a rule, American evangelists had not been warmly received in that country.

But the moment we prayed for the sick and miracles began to take place, indifference vanished. During those few weeks, we proved to ourselves that the ministry of miracles was needed to evangelize the world. Night after night, every kind of miracle took place. The deaf heard and the blind saw by the scores. People who were brought in totally paralyzed, rose from their beds and leaped for joy. As a result of these miracles, great numbers turned to the Lord. We returned to America persuaded that the ministry of miracles would revolutionize evangelism on mission fields. We were convinced that God would confirm His Word with signs following. We were certain it was the will of God for us to claim His promises.

To discover God's will in prayer, accept His revealed will. Where God has made His will plain through His Word, reverently accept it without question. When He has not made His will clear, then pray like Christ, "Not my will but thine be done."

CHAPTER VII

The Secret of Daily Contact

Give us day by day our daily bread (Lk. 11:3).

These words contain another vital secret in the art of praying to change things — the principle of daily contact with the living God. Jesus taught us to pray, "Give us day by day our daily bread."

God has ordained certain laws to govern His universe. In no sphere is the immutableness of these laws more evident than in the realm of prayer. Successful prayer requires daily contact with God. When a person's spiritual life begins to deteriorate, it can generally be traced to a lack of consistent daily prayer. It is amazing to learn the small amount of time many people, even ministers, give to real prayer. Perhaps they spend five or ten minutes a day in prayer, and then they are on their way. No wonder the forces of darkness mobilize against them and in some cases, completely paralyze their efforts.

A successful life is shaped in the crucible of the daily hour of prayer. God must work with the material given Him. If there is little material available, He is limited in what He can do. Many people do not realize there is actual substance to prayer. God stores up the prayers of His saints to use at the proper time (Rev. 8:3). The prayers of God's people are used in a vital way to execute His plan on earth.

God has ordained for us to have the resources of heaven at our command. Jesus said, "All authority has been given to Me in heaven and on earth" (Matt. 28:18). "Go into all the world and preach the gospel to every creature" (Mk. 16:15). "As the Father has sent Me, I also send you" (Jn. 20:21). The Church can undertake this momentous task because all power has been made available. But it is available only to those who keep in contact with their God daily.

"Give us day by day our daily bread." Jesus did not ask us to pray for a year's, or a month's, or even a week's supply of bread. God wants us daily to depend on Him. He wants us to daily recognize the need of His presence and His sustaining power.

THE DAILY MANNA

Daily dependence on God was taught in the giving of manna to the children of Israel. They were to receive only enough for a day's supply. No man could gather a supply and hoard it for future use. Those who did found it bred worms and was unfit for human consumption.

Many Christians would rather have healing they can't "lose" than health that comes from a daily dependence on the quickening power of the Spirit of God. They would rather have financial security than daily go to the secret chamber and ask God to meet their needs. They would like a baptism in the Holy Ghost that does not require daily waiting on God for a fresh anointing. But these desires are not in accordance with God's purpose.

God's plan involves daily dependence on Him. Without Him you can do nothing. To successfully accomplish His will, you must not allow a single day to pass without communion with God. "Man shall not live by bread alone, but by every word that proceeds from the mouth of God" (Matt. 4:4). Just as the body feels the effect of going without food, so the spirit suffers when it is not fed the Bread of Life.

Daniel is an excellent example of one who learned the secret of true success. His life spanned a century, during which time dynasties rose and fell. It was one of the most turbulent eras in the history of the world. Time and again Daniel's life was in jeopardy. Once he was condemned to die with all the wise men of Babylon. At another time, he was thrown into a den of vicious lions. On each occasion, his life was miraculously preserved.

Daniel's integrity and wisdom caused him to rise in favor with each succeeding regime. Because the Spirit of God dwelt in him, he was admired and respected by kings and queens (Dan. 5:11). Whenever an emergency arose, they turned to him for help. For the better part of a century his life influenced nations. His fearless courage and faith moved kings to acknowledge the true God.

What was the secret to Daniel's power? Prayer was a priority with him. He did not go running to God just when some crisis appeared. Crises were common in his life, but when they came he always knew what to do. Three times a day he met with God and gave thanks. He allowed nothing to interrupt his daily habit.

Jealous men schemed to take Daniel's life by convincing King Darius to for thirty days forbid the petitioning of any god or any man — except the king. Anyone who violated the order would be thrown into a pit with lions. But Daniel did not panic — He continued worshiping God as usual. "Now when Daniel knew that the writing was signed, he went home. And in his upper room, with his windows open toward Jerusalem, he knelt down on his knees three times that day, and prayed and gave thanks before his God, as was his custom since early days" (Dan. 6:10). Here was Daniel's secret: Daily prayer. Kingdoms might rise and fall and wicked men conspire against his life, but he knew in Whom he believed.

DANIEL MOVES A "MOUNTAIN"

When he was young, Daniel — along with many others — had been carried away from Jerusalem by the King of Babylon. This tragedy caused him great sorrow. When he opened his window toward Jerusalem to pray every day, his thoughts were with his people who suffered under the heavy hand of divine chastisement.

How he longed to see their restoration. But first a "mountain" would have to be moved. The destructive "mountain" of Babylon held the Israelites in subjection and would not let them go. But Daniel believed that God could move that mountain. He committed himself to prayer and fasting. "Then I set my face toward the Lord God to make request by prayer and supplications, with fasting, sackcloth, and ashes" (Dan. 9:3). And Babylon was moved! God raised up King Cyrus to accomplish His purpose (Isa. 44:28). Cyrus overthrew the Babylonian kingdom, and shortly after decreed the restoration of Jerusalem. Jeremiah 51:24,25 speaks of God moving the "destroying mountain" so that Daniel's people might return to Jerusalem.

> "And I will repay Babylon and all the inhabitants of Chaldea for all the evil they have done in Zion in your sight," says the LORD. "Behold, I am against you, *O destroying mountain*, who destroys all the earth," says the LORD. "*And I will stretch out My hand against you, roll you down from the rocks, and make you a burnt mountain*" (Jer. 51:24,25).

And so the "mountain" was moved! As far as we know, Daniel's prayers never failed to receive an answer, though sometimes it seemed doubtful. There were occasions when Satan fiercely contested Daniel's claim on God's promise. Once the powers of darkness battled against him for 21 days. But he never wavered, and in the end, the battle turned to victory. The regularity of Daniel's prayer kept the devil from having a chance to get a wedge in. Daniel proved that a man could live for a whole century in victory!

The mighty effect of daily prayer is revealed in Christ's life. He did not allow anything to interfere with His regular communion with God. Sometimes it was necessary for Him to rise early in the morning to have His time of prayer before the people started coming to Him. When a great decision was to be made, He would seclude himself in a remote place where He could spend hours in prayer. He knew prayer was the only way He could accomplish His great purpose.

THE LESSON OF THE BREACHED WALLS

The importance of meeting daily with God in earnest prayer is forcefully illustrated by the following story:

A Christian Armenian merchant was transporting merchandise by caravan across the desert to a town in Turkish Armenia. He was raised in a Christian home and daily committed himself into the hands of God.

At the time, the country was infested with Kurds — bandits who robbed caravans. Unknown to the merchant, these bandits had been following his caravan, intending to rob it at the first camping place on the plains.

After dark, at the designated time the Kurds drew close to the camp. Everything was strangely quiet — no guards or watchmen. But as they came nearer, to their astonishment they saw high walls standing around the caravan.

They tried again the next night, and found the same impassable walls. On the third night, the walls were standing but there were broken places through which the Kurds could enter.

Terrified by the mystery, the captain of the Kurds awakened the merchant. "What does this mean? Ever since you left Ezerum, we followed, intending to rob you. The first and second night, we found high walls around the caravan, but tonight, we entered through broken places. If you will tell us the secret behind this, I will not harm you."

The merchant, himself, was surprised and puzzled. "My friends," he said, "I have done nothing to raise the walls around us. All I do is pray every evening, committing myself and those with me to God. I fully trust in Him to keep me from all evil. But tonight, because I was very tired and sleepy, I made a rather half-hearted prayer. That must be why you were allowed to break through!"

The Kurds were overwhelmed by this testimony. Immediately, they gave their lives to Jesus Christ, and were saved. From caravan robbers, they became God-fearing men. And the Armenian merchant never forgot the breach in the wall of prayer.

Here is another secret of mighty prayer: To move mountains, prayer must be a lifestyle. The one who wants answers to his prayers must, like Daniel, regularly meet with God. Prayer must become as natural as breathing. Through prayer, spiritual forces that human efforts cannot overcome will be defeated. By continuous prayer, the enemy is kept at bay and a hedge of protection keeps evil from penetrating it.

CHAPTER VIII

The Secret of the Blood of the Covenant

And forgive us our debts, as we forgive our debtors (Matt. 6:12).

But into the second part the high priest went alone once a year, not without blood, which he offered for himself and for the people's sins committed in ignorance ... But Christ came as High Priest of the good things to come ... with His own blood He entered the Most Holy Place once for all, having obtained eternal redemption (Heb. 9:7,11,12).

Let us therefore come boldly to the throne of grace, that we may obtain mercy and find grace to help in time of need (Heb. 4:16).

Jesus continued His instructions on prayer with the words, "And forgive us our debts, as we forgive our debtors." In approaching the throne of grace, one must have assurance that his sins are forgiven. Yet many pray not knowing this and wonder why their prayers go unanswered. How can someone approach a holy God with unforgiven sin? How can they claim help from heaven when they are in rebellion against God?

There is a way, however! God in His great love made provision through the blood of the covenant. In the Old Testament, people could not directly approach God. They did not dare go into the Holy of Holies where the Divine Presence dwelt. Once a year, the high priest went into the sacred place to offer blood for the atonement of the sins of the people. But the method was faulty. A priest had to stand between God and the people and this act of atonement had to be repeated every year. *But Christ has changed all this. He has entered the Holy of Holies with His own blood — once and for all — making atonement for the whole human race.* Therefore, the believer can receive forgiveness for sin through the blood of Jesus, and with boldness approach the throne of grace!

ISRAEL'S PRAYERS WERE DENIED

Many pray in ignorance, without first asking God to forgive their sins. The prayer which should come before all others is, "God be merciful to me a sinner."

Although every Christian knows he sins, not all ask forgiveness. Unconfessed sin is the reason that some Christians' prayers are not answered. It is useless to try and move mountains if sin stands in the way.

When Israel, God's chosen people, fell into apostasy, they wondered why their prayers were not being answered. The prophet Isaiah cried out, "Behold, the Lord's hand is not shortened, that it cannot save; nor His ear heavy, that it cannot hear. But your iniquities have separated you from your God; and your sins have hidden His face from you, so that He will not hear" (Isa. 59:1,2). Sin will always stand in the way of mountains being moved.

CONFESSION — THE SECRET TO PRAYER THAT BRINGS REVIVAL

Confession is a very important element in prayer — not just for those praying the sinner's prayer for salvation, but for Christians. In studying biblical accounts, those who confessed their sins and failures had the most power with God.

Not a single thing is recorded against Daniel's conduct. Yet his confession of sin if one of the deepest on record. In Daniel 9, we find the prophet confessing the sins of his people as his own:

1. We have sinned.
2. We have committed iniquity.
3. We have been wicked.
4. We have rebelled against God.
5. We have departed from His precepts.
6. We have not listened to His servants.
7. Our princes and all the people of the land have not heeded His servants.

It was during this time of confession that the angel Gabriel appeared to Daniel and showed him the vision of seventy weeks. This revealed to Daniel that his people would soon return from captivity and rebuild Jerusalem as well as the time Israel's Messiah was to appear!

While Job sat in ashes grieving over his tribulations, he questioned God's wisdom. But when he repented, God healed him and blessed the latter part of his life even more than He had the first.

It was when Isaiah cried out, "I am undone" (Isa. 6:5), that a live coal was taken from the altar and put on his lips. He proceeded to write one of the greatest books ever written.

When David confessed his sin, the Lord had mercy on him. David found pardon and restoration when he said to God, "I acknowledge my transgressions, and my sin is ever before me. Against You, You only, have I sinned, and done this evil in Your sight" (Psa. 51:3,4).

God heard even wicked Ahab, husband of the notorious Jezebel, when he humbled himself before God (I Ki. 21:27-29).

The devil is the accuser of the brethren. One way for Christians to stay one step ahead of him is to confess sin before he has a chance to accuse them.

Many of the world's greatest revivals occurred when people mourned before God and confessed their sins. When the city of Nineveh was about to be destroyed, the inhabitants — from the king on down — put on sackcloth and humbled themselves before God, and He spared their city.

The story of the Finney revivals is a dramatic one. This move of God was undoubtedly the most significant in America during the nineteenth century. In Finney's autobiography, he relates many instances of powerful revivals occurring after Christians broke down before God and repented of their lukewarmness.

Jonathan's Goforth's book *By My Spirit*, records remarkable revivals in China during the early part of the twentieth century. In his narrative, Mr. Goforth showed that these revivals were born out of Christians earnestly searching their hearts.

When Christians are broken over their sins and are willing to confess and forsake them, revival reaches its greatest power and purity. One of the most striking elements of the Azuza Street revival were the copious tears shed by those who knelt at the altars in that humble building.

Confession and repentance of sin are the only things that will save America. Self-judgment must begin at the house of God. There is no doubt if the Church would repent of her prayerlessness and lack of passion for souls, she would give tremendous impetus to this last-day revival. When we bare our souls before God, we can expect to see our prayers answered.

A WORD OF CAUTION

At this point, let me give a word of caution. Satan will try one way or another to trick people. Some believers have an overactive conscience, and continually dig up their old sins after they have repented and God has forgotten them. Often these people despair of ever having divine forgiveness. They need to be directed to God's promise that the darkest sin can be washed away by the blood of Jesus. God has promised that He will remember our sins no more

(Jer. 31:34). If God no longer remembers, neither should we. It is the work of the devil to accuse those whose sins are under the blood.

However, if your prayers are not being answered, and you do not know why, you should pray as the Psalmist, "Search me, O God, and know my heart; Try me, and know my anxieties; and see if there is any wicked way in me" (Psa. 139:23,24).

Perhaps restitution needs to be made. Restitution is clearly taught in the Old Testament (Lev. 5:15,16). We also see a striking illustration of this in the New Testament story of Zaccheus. Zaccheus, a despised publican whose method of gathering taxes was a national scandal, was paid a visit by Jesus. Zaccheus knew he was wrong and was ready to make restitution. He said to the Lord, "Look, Lord, I give half of my goods to the poor; and if I have taken anything from anyone by false accusation, I restore fourfold" (Lk. 19:8). And Jesus responded by saying, "Today salvation has come to this house" (Lk. 19:9).

IDOLS AND UNANSWERED PRAYER

Some do not receive answers to their prayers because they unknowingly have idols. Anything that displaces God for first place in one's life is an idol. The great commandment is to love the Lord with all our hearts, soul and mind. To be devoted to anything more than to God is a violation of that commandment. Whatever we love more than God — money, popularity, home or family — becomes an idol. The Lord said to Ezekiel concerning the elders who had inquired of Him:

> Son of man, these men have set up their idols in their hearts, and put before them that which causes them to stumble into iniquity. Should I let Myself be inquired of at all by them? (Ezek. 14:3).

God did not hear the prayers of men who retained idols in their hearts. To have influence with God, a person must put Him before everything else.

There are many things that can hold back answers to prayer. Failure to properly provide for your family, for instance. The Bible says that person is worse than an unbeliever (I Tim. 5:8). Some husbands support their family well, but save all their courtesy for those outside the home. This is also true of some wives. Their ugly disposition and disagreeable conduct at home defies their profession of faith. Such inconsideration may hinder prayers from reaching God.

> Likewise you husbands, dwell with them with understanding, giving honor to the wife, as to the weaker vessel, and as being heirs together of the grace of life, that *your prayers may not be hindered* (I Pet. 3:7).

Here is the reason for many unanswered prayers: Unconfessed sin. If you want miracles in your life, supernatural answers to prayer, or if a mountain is holding back your progress and needs to be moved, then confess and forsake the sin that may be standing between you and God.

CHAPTER IX

The Secret Hindrance to Prayer

And forgive us our debts, As we forgive our debtors (Matt. 6:12).

For assuredly, I say to you, whoever says to this mountain, "Be removed and be cast into the sea," and does not doubt in his heart, but believes that those things he says will come to pass, he will have whatever he says. ... And whenever you stand praying, if you have anything against anyone, forgive him, that your Father in heaven may also forgive you your trespasses. But if you do not forgive, neither will your Father in heaven forgive your trespasses (Mk. 11:23,25,26).

The Lord declared that the prayer of faith would cause mountains to be rooted up and cast into the sea. But He also spoke of a condition, which if not met, could not only hinder the fulfillment of such a prayer, but also could be the cause of one being denied divine forgiveness.

Jesus said in Matthew 6:14,15, "For if you forgive men their trespasses, your heavenly Father will also forgive you. But if you do not forgive men their trespasses, neither will your Father forgive your trespasses." Has God forgiven us? The answer is clear. To the extent we forgive others, we are forgiven!

Here is a matter of crucial importance in the art of praying to change things. Jesus announced that prayer could move a mighty mountain from its foundations and hurl it into the depths of the sea. Yet such a prayer can be lawfully prayed only by those who freely "forgive their debtors." If you don't, all your praying is vain. Prayer from an unforgiving heart will never be accepted at the throne of grace. This is a difficult lesson for some people to learn. There are people who have developed a bitter spirit from being wronged or thinking they have been wronged. Bitterness in your heart makes it absolutely impossible for your prayers to be answered. Allowing bitterness to take hold of you, makes you a victim of your anger toward another.

Even if people conduct themselves so that they can no longer be fully trusted, our forgiveness of them must always be generous and complete. We dare not retain even the smallest part of bitterness. Such an attitude will disease our own soul, as well as deprive us of access to the throne of grace.

SEVENTY TIMES SEVEN

Peter was of the opinion that there should be a limit to forgiveness. He had asked, "Lord, how often shall my brother sin against me, and I forgive him? Up to seven times?" (Matt. 18:21). Jesus answered, "I do not say to you, up to seven times, but up to seventy times seven" (Matt. 18:22). And before Peter could recover from the shock, Jesus related the parable of the unforgiving servant. This servant owed ten thousand talents, but was unable to pay. He begged his master for mercy. Because the master was compassionate, he granted forgiveness for the entire debt.

But this servant found a fellow servant who owed him a hundred denarii. He had no mercy on him. He took him by the throat, and demanded he pay up. But the man could not, and the evil servant threw him into prison. When the master heard what happened, he gave orders for the servant who showed no mercy to be sent to prison until he had paid all. Jesus then added, "So My heavenly Father also will do to you if each of you, from his heart, does not forgive his brother his trespasses" (Matt. 18:35).

Jesus practiced what He preached. After He was beaten at the whipping post, mocked by the crowd, crowned with thorns, and nailed to the cross to suffer hours in excruciating agony, He looked up to His heavenly Father and prayed for His enemies: "Father, forgive them, for they do not know what they do" (Lk. 23:34).

The great wonder of redemption is that there is mercy for the sinner — for those who deserve no mercy. But to obtain God's mercy, a person must be merciful. When Christ said that mountains could be moved by the prayer of faith, He qualified that great promise with a certain condition — the willingness to forgive.

If you say to a mountain, "Be removed and be cast into the sea" (Mk 11:23), you must also have grace to say to those who have sinned against you, "I freely forgive you." Most Christians understand the importance of a forgiving spirit, but few place the emphasis Christ did. He made it an absolute condition to the answering of prayer. Why did He place such great importance upon it? Because those who exercise forgiveness can only do so by having the love of God in their hearts. Only the ones who have His kind of love are worthy to move mountains. As Paul said, "And though I have all faith, so that I could remove mountains, but have not love (divine love), I am nothing" (I Cor. 13:2).

In His Sermon on the Mount, Christ showed the importance of believers maintaining a right relationship with other believers. If someone came to the altar with their gift, and remembered their brother had something against them, they were to leave the gift at the altar and immediately go and seek reconciliation. Afterward, they could return and offer their gift (Matt. 5:23,24). Failure to seek reconciliation with other members of the body of Christ is a serious offense against the principles of divine government. Those refusing reconciliation with their brother were to be treated as though they were heathen (Matt. 18:17).

One of the most beautiful illustrations of forgiveness is found in the story of Joseph. Few have ever been treated worse by their own brothers than Joseph was. As a young boy, he was sold into slavery by his own brothers, and carried captive into a foreign land. There he was subjected to severe trials and temptations. Because of a false and malicious accusation, he was thrown into prison to suffer for two long years. Eventually the time came when he was in a position to execute full retribution on his brothers who had showed him no mercy. Instead he chose to extend kindness to them for their evil, and in so doing, he received divine blessing above all others (Gen. 49:22-26).

God has promised that the prayer of faith will move mountains. But those who claim the promise must have a forgiving spirit. In order to say to the mountain, "Be removed and be cast into the sea" (Mk. 11:23), you must also say to any who have wronged you, "I freely forgive you."

CHAPTER X

The Secret of Prayer That Anticipates Evil

Then the devil, taking Him up on a high mountain, showed Him all the kingdoms of the world in a moment of time. And the devil said to Him, "All this authority I will give You, and their glory; for this has been delivered to me, and I give it to whomever I wish. Therefore, if You will worship before me, all will be Yours" (Lk. 4:5-7).

And do not lead us into temptation, but deliver us from the evil one. For Yours is the kingdom and the power and the glory forever. Amen (Matt. 6:13).

Prayer can move mountains. But to pray this prayer, we must also be willing to meet and overcome the temptations involved. Christ was taken up to a high mountain, where He received a dazzling offer from the prince of this world (Lk. 4:5-7). From the vantage point of the mountain, the devil showed Jesus the kingdoms of this world and their glory. He then proposed to give all to Jesus if He would only fall down and worship him. Christ rejected the devil's offer, declaring worship was for God only.

Mountains have often been the place of the testing for saints. At Mt. Sinai, the children of Israel witnessed awe-inspiring thundering and lightning. This scene caused them to draw back and say to Moses, "You speak with us, and we will hear; but let not God speak with us, lest we die" (Ex. 20:19). But Moses replied, "'Do not fear; for God has come to test you, and that His fear may be before you, so that you may not sin'" (Ex. 20:20).

On Mt. Moriah Abraham met the supreme test of his life: He was asked to give up his only son, Isaac. "By faith Abraham, when he was tested, offered up Isaac ... accounting that God was able to raise him up, even from the dead" (Heb. 11:17,19). Abraham's steadfastness in meeting the test caused him to be called father of the faithful (see Gal. 3:6-9).

On Mt. Carmel, Elijah challenged the prophets of Baal and called Israel back to God with the words, "How long will you falter between two opinions? If the LORD is God, follow Him; but if Baal, then follow him" (I Ki. 18:21). Elijah's faith in his God was justified when in answer to his prayer, fire came down from heaven and burned up the sacrifice.

To move mountains, you must be willing to meet the challenge. You must be able to scale the mountain's height and take its measurement. And always, the higher one climbs, the greater the temptations will be. At the top, you will meet the tempter face to face as Christ met him. And sooner or later, you will face the devil's more subtle temptation — pride and ambition. Satan, knowing that Christ had successfully overcome all other temptations, gave Him one more — the promise that all the kingdoms of the world would be His, if He would worship him.

THE SECRET OF VICTORY OVER TEMPTATION

All must face temptation, just as Christ did. But it is foolish to put oneself in the way of temptation. That is why Christ taught us to pray, "And do not lead us into temptation, but deliver us from the evil one." *This is praying with anticipation evil. It allows for deliverance from evil before it can even reach us!*

A young Christian mother learned the secret of God's protecting guidance. Prayer had become a very important part in her life and she became sensitive to the Holy Spirit's leading. Daily living in the

Spirit resulted in praying in time to avert tragedy in the life of her child. This is her testimony:

> One fall day, just before school was to be let out, a great fear suddenly gripped my heart. Something tragic was about to happen. I knew that one of my children was in danger. This was a new experience for me, as I knew only happiness since I had been saved. I realized this was a warning from God, so I began to pray. Relief came and a great calm came over me. I rose up, thanking the Lord.

> When I saw my children running down the road, I stepped out of the gate to meet them. As they came near, one of the girls reported that our neighbor's little boy had been struck by a car.

> My little boy, Johnny, came up with a puzzled expression on his face. He said, "Mother, that car would have gotten me too, for we were crossing the road together, but it was going so fast that the wind from the car just picked me up and set me out of the road." I told him it was the hand of God that moved him from the path of danger.

SOME PRAYERS ARE PRAYED TOO LATE

Some people seek God earnestly after they get into trouble, not realizing that had they prayed sooner, they might have avoided the pitfall. It is best to foresee evil and avoid it. "A prudent man foresees evil and hides himself; the simple pass on and are punished" (Prov. 27:12). How can we hope to escape the traps the devil continually sets? The answer lies not in human foresight or wisdom. "Trust in the LORD with all your heart, and lean not on your own understanding" (Prov. 3:5).

There is a place of safety. This place of safety and protection from evil is plainly revealed in the 91st Psalm:

> He who dwells in the secret place of the Most High shall abide under the shadow of the Almighty. ... Surely He shall deliver you from the snare of the fowler and from the

perilous pestilence. He shall cover you with His feathers, and under His wings you shall take refuge (Psa. 91:1,3,4).

This is a promise for deliverance from Satan's traps! The expression "snare of the fowler" refers to the work of Satan, who is busy setting snares for God's people. Many get caught in Satan's snares and sometimes God in His mercy somehow extricates them. But how much better to be aware and avoid the snares. Jesus taught believers to pray to be delivered from evil rather than to be rescued from it after it engulfs them.

The lesson of anticipating temptation, is clearly portrayed in the drama of Gethsemane. There, Jesus met the greatest crisis of His life. The powers of darkness concentrated their forces in a desperate effort to defeat the purpose of God with one overwhelming attack on Christ. As Jesus prayed that fateful night, His soul was in excruciating pain. "Sweat ... like great drops of blood" (Lk. 22:44) fell to the ground. Jesus wrestled on in agonizing prayer while His disciples slept. Though Jesus had told them to pray that they would not fall into temptation, they were apparently ignorant of the drama that was engaging the attention of the universe.

They too, were about to meet the greatest crisis of their lives. Soon the betrayer would appear and they would be thrown into panic and confusion. And they would not be prepared because when they could have followed Christ's instructions to fortify themselves against the storm that lay ahead, they slept.

The disciples slept right up until the armed soldiers came. They awoke to great confusion. One of them struck the High Priest's slave and cut off his ear. After Jesus' arrest, Peter, in panic, spoke before he thought, only to discover that he had denied his Lord. He wept bitterly over his act of cowardice. What he wouldn't give to turn time back just a few hours. His great mistake was failing to pray when temptation threatened. He did not heed Jesus' warning to "rise and pray." Instead he slept on while his world was falling apart.

A WARNING FOR OUR TIME

Jesus' warning to watch and pray was not for the disciples alone. The warning is applicable to all Christians, and especially for those who live in the time just preceding His return. When Jesus gave His great discourse on the events prior to His second coming, He warned that the "cares of this life" would cause that day to come upon many "unexpectedly" (Lk. 21:34). "For it will come as a snare on all those who dwell on the face of the whole earth" (Lk. 21:35). He gave a special warning to those who would live in that day:

> Watch therefore, and pray always that you may be counted worthy to escape all these things that will come to pass, and to stand before the Son of Man (Lk. 21:36).

So Jesus warned that the only way to escape the pitfalls peculiar to the last hours of this age was to "watch and pray always." To those who would, He gave the great promise of Revelation 3:10:

> Because you have kept My command to persevere, I also will keep you from the hour of trial which shall come upon the whole world, to test those who dwell on the earth.

Anticipating evil and avoiding it by seeking the Lord's counsel is repeatedly taught in the Scriptures. In Joshua's day, the children of Israel had won some notable victories. However, they were tricked into making a pact with the Gibeonites that they would not kill them. They fell into a trap simply because in the midst of victory, they neglected to ask counsel of the Lord (Josh. 9:14). Centuries later, because Saul went against the treaty made earlier and killed some of the Gibeonites, judgment came on Saul's household (II Sam. 21:1).

In David's wanderings in the wilderness, the hand of God intervened and preserved him many times. That was because David was wise, he made it a habit to inquire of the Lord before each move. One time, Saul came to besiege David and his men at Keilah, a city where they were living temporarily. David had reason to feel secure in that city, because he and his men had saved it from the Philistines.

But David asked the Lord about the situation and was warned that the citizens would betray him. So he and his men left Keilah at once (I Sam. 23:5-11).

Nehemiah was a mighty man of prayer. His enemies opposed him and ridiculed his work. At one point, they bribed someone to try to persuade him to hide because of a supposed plot to kill him. But God revealed to Nehemiah that the whole scheme was fraudulent, and was intended to discredit him in the eyes of the people (Neh. 6). Nehemiah was a man who knew how to avoid the traps of the enemy because he was a man of prayer.

God's plan for His children is that they anticipate temptation and avoid it. Jesus taught men to pray, "Do not lead us into temptation, but deliver us from the evil one." Christians must constantly watch and pray so they do not enter into temptation. That is better than having to ask God to rescue them out of trouble.

CHAPTER XI

The Secret of Receiving Financial Blessings

> But when you do a charitable deed, do not let your left hand
> know what your right hand is doing, that your charitable
> deed may be in secret; and your Father who sees in secret
> will Himself reward you openly (Matt. 6:3,4).

These words were spoken by Jesus as He began His great lesson
on prayer. Giving is vitally related to receiving. God's purpose for
our receiving abundantly is that we may give abundantly. To make
the lesson even more emphatic, Jesus concluded with an admonition
against unnecessarily storing up material wealth. He said:

> Do not lay up for yourselves treasures on earth, where
> moth and rust destroy and where thieves break in and
> steal; but lay up for yourselves treasures in heaven,
> where neither moth nor rust destroys and where thieves
> do not break in and steal (Matt. 6:19,20).

The secret to abundant receiving requires learning the art of
abundant giving. Jesus said, "Freely you have received, freely give"
(Matt. 10:8). Those who freely give will freely receive.

> Give, and it will be given to you: good measure, pressed
> down, shaken together, and running over will be put into
> your bosom. For with the same measure that you use, it
> will be measured back to you (Lk. 6:38).

We must take note that God often answers our prayers by moving on the hearts of others. George Mueller maintained his orphanages by the generous gifts of others. Mueller was a man with a burden of caring for 2,000 children. People were amazed at what God did for Mueller. They didn't understand how he could have peace of mind with such a responsibility. What if the needed funds failed to come in? What if the large number of children should suddenly be in want? Would not God's work suffer reproach? But what was needed always came in. Though on occasions Mueller was severely tried, the required answer always arrived in time. God's Spirit moved on someone's heart just at the right moment. God not only provided him with the means to support orphans, but also with funds to accomplish a worldwide mission work. Mueller received much, but he also gave much.

Here is where many fail. They want God to give to them, they want Him to move mountains, but they are stingy when it comes to giving to God. This is true of many who have received healing. They take advantage of God. Though they have spent thousands of dollars on medical treatment without receiving permanent help, when God heals them, they don't even give a tithe to the Lord on the amount they spent previously.

I believe people withhold from God because of unbelief and uncertainty of the future. They fear that God may fail them later on and reason that it would be best to accumulate a large reserve just in case. God is not against a person making proper provision for his family, but as believers, we must do the same for God's work. Those who can't trust God for their needs, both present and future, have no faith that God answers prayer. Faith requires action. Giving is an act of faith. And it is the insurance of continued receiving.

Nearly every person who has been greatly used of God was asked by God to give up all. They were placed in a position where, in the natural, there was no security. Some gave up a prosperous business, a responsible position, or even a relationship.

Abraham faced such a trial when God asked him to sacrifice his son Isaac. To be Christ's disciples, we must be willing to give up all. God wants to know which we prize most — eternal or temporal things.

HOW TO RECEIVE 100-FOLD

The rich young ruler was tested regarding his values. He came to Jesus asking what to do to receive eternal life. Jesus' answer staggered him.

> One thing you lack: Go your way, sell whatever you have and give to the poor, and you will have treasure in heaven; and come, take up the cross, and follow Me (Mk. 10:21).

The young man went away sorrowful, "for he had great possessions" (Mk. 10:22). Many have preached that it would have been better for the young man to have followed Jesus, even if it meant dying in poverty. But such a conclusion is not necessarily correct. When the young ruler left, Peter rather sadly remarked that they had left all to follow Jesus. The Lord turned to him and made a strange remark — so strange few people believe it. He said:

> There is no one who has left house or brothers or sisters or father or mother or wife or children or lands, for My sake and the gospel's, *who shall not receive a hundred-fold* now in this time — houses and brothers and sisters and mothers and children *and lands*, with persecutions — and in the age to come, eternal life (Mk. 10:29,30).

Yes, Jesus said that if someone left houses and lands, they would receive "a hundredfold now in this time" — including houses and lands. Besides that, eternal life in the world to come. But first, we must prove we want eternal life more than all the houses and lands in the world. We demonstrate our faith by our willingness to give all we have to God, regardless of the outcome.

Christ never disapproved of people giving, even when they had little to give. Not long after His encounter with the young ruler,

Christ saw a widow drop two mites into the offering box of the temple. He commended her, pointing out that she had given more than everyone because she had given "her whole livelihood" (Mk. 12:44). It was a great act of faith on her part, and according to the law of giving and receiving that Jesus taught, it was also an act of wisdom.

THE SECRET OF POWER IN THE EARLY CHURCH

Those in the Early Church knew how to get their prayers answered. When Peter was in prison awaiting execution, the prayers of the Christians sent an angel to open the prison. Every day God's mighty power was revealed in the Jerusalem Church. Signs, wonders and miracles were common occurrences. People came from surrounding cities to be healed, and "they were all healed" (Acts. 5:16).

Many people wonder why that same power for healing is not present today. The answer may be found in the context. When the believers in the Early Church accepted Christ, they gave all — their homes and their possessions. This provided the means necessary for evangelizing that generation. They called nothing their own.

> Now the multitude of those who believed were of one heart and one soul; neither did anyone say that any of the things he possessed was his own, but they had all things in common. And with great power the apostles gave witness to the resurrection of the Lord Jesus. And great grace was upon them all (Acts 4:32,33).

JACOB'S EXPERIENCE

Jacob had faith, but his besetting sin was covetousness. His concept of religion caused him to try to see how much he could get out of it. His trickery finally resulted in his being forced to leave everything and flee for his life. While in flight, he had the opportunity to reflect on the results of his scheming. With this on his mind, he spent a night at Bethel. There he had a vision of a ladder to heaven with angels of God passing up and down. This glimpse of another world changed his whole life. When he awoke from his vision, he promised God that from then on, he would give a tenth of all.

> Then Jacob made a vow, saying, "If God will be with me, and keep me in this way that I am going, and give me bread to eat and clothing to put on, so that I come back to my father's house in peace, then the LORD shall be my God. ... And of all that You give me I will surely give a tenth to You" (Gen. 28:20-22).

It was hard for Jacob to change his ways, but God helped and blessed him. The great crisis of Jacob's life occurred years later when Esau rode with 400 men of war to attack him. That night, Jacob wrestled with God and prevailed. Esau, who had wanted to kill him, instead threw his arms around Jacob and wept. Esau had found that his cheating brother had changed. He was no longer Jacob, but Israel — a prince with God.

THE STORY OF THE KERR GLASS MANUFACTURING COMPANY THAT SURVIVED THE QUAKE

The Scripture which relates Jacob's covenant with God made a great impression upon Alexander H. Kerr, who was converted under D.L. Moody. He saw that Jacob had nothing when he made that promise to God, but twenty years later, he returned home with great abundance. In June 1902, Mr. Kerr made a special covenant to set aside a certain percentage of his income for the work of the Lord. At the time, he was poor, having a mortgage on his home and many financial obligations.

That same year, with very small capital, Mr. Kerr organized in San Francisco the firm known as the Kerr Glass Manufacturing Company. It was to become one of the largest firms selling fruit jars in the United States.

Mr. Kerr had put practically every cent he had into this fruit jar enterprise. Then the San Francisco earthquake came! His friends told him he was a ruined man. He replied, "I don't believe it; or if I am, then the Bible is not true. I know God will not go back on His promises." He wired to San Francisco, and received the following reply: "Your factory is in the heart of the fire, and undoubtedly is destroyed. The heat is so intense, we will be unable to find out anything for some days."

What a time of testing! But his faith in the Lord never wavered. He believed Malachi 3:11, and stood firm on this promise. About a week after the earthquake and fire, a second telegram arrived saying, "Everything for a mile and a half on all sides of the factory burned; but your factory was miraculously saved."

The factory was a two-storied wooden building, containing huge tanks — kept at 2,500 degrees — where glass was melted, and oil was used for fuel. This building was probably the most flammable in San Francisco. The fire had raged on all sides of this glass factory, creeping up to the wooden fence surrounding it, even leaping over and scorching it. The flames went beyond the building, burning everything in its path. However, neither the building nor the wooden fence surrounding it, were burned. Not a single glass jar was cracked by the earthquake or fire!

The apostle John said in I John 3:22: "And whatever we ask we receive from Him, because we keep His commandments and do those things that are pleasing in His sight." The context refers to giving: "But whoever has this world's goods, and sees his brother in need, and shuts up his heart from him, how does the love of God abide in him?" (I Jn. 3:17). When believers see the millions dying without Christ, and refuse to give liberally to reach them with the Gospel of deliverance, can they expect to have their prayers abundantly answered? The law of giving and receiving is nowhere expressed more clearly than in the well-known verse in Malachi 3:10:

"Bring all the tithes into the storehouse, that there may be food in My house, and prove Me now in this," says the LORD of hosts, "If I will not open for you the windows of heaven and pour out for you such blessing that there will not be room enough to receive it."

The law of giving and receiving is a law invariable in its operation as the law of gravity. Do you want your prayers answered? Do you want to receive abundantly from God? Do you want financial blessings? Then "give, and it will be given to you: good measure, pressed down, shaken together, and running over will be put into your bosom. For with the same measure that you use, it will be measured back to you" (Lk. 6:38).

CHAPTER XII

The Secret to Increasing Power in Prayer 10-Fold

Assuredly, I say to you, whatever you bind on earth will be bound in heaven, and whatever you loose on earth will be loosed in heaven. Again I say to you that if two of you agree on earth concerning anything that they ask, it will be done for them by My Father in heaven (Matt. 18:18,19).

Now we come to another very important secret in the art of praying to change things — the power of agreement. In Matthew 18, Christ mentioned His Church and dealt with the issue of unity. He gave special instructions for preserving that unity (Matt. 18:15-17). Then He climaxed His teaching by showing the great power available when believers pray together with one purpose and mind.

THE 10-FOLD INCREASE OF POWER

Mighty as the prayer of one individual can be, it cannot be compared with the possible results when two or more pray in agreement. There is strength in unity. This strength is compounded in the spiritual realm. Joshua said to the children of Israel, "One man of you shall chase a thousand ..." (Josh. 23:10). But Moses declared that "two put ten thousand to flight" (Deut. 32:30). *The power of two agreeing in prayer increases tenfold over one!*

God knows that working together His Church can accomplish much more than individuals working independently. If the Church is to accomplish her great purpose, all members must work in proper relation to each other. When the members of the body of Christ pray in absolute agreement, their prayers will cause mountains to move.

Just before Christ's ascension to heaven, He told His disciples to wait in Jerusalem "for the Promise of the Father ... for John truly baptized with water, but you shall be baptized with the Holy Spirit not many days from now" (Acts 1:4,5). In obedience to this command, the disciples returned to Jerusalem and "continued with one accord in prayer and supplication" (Acts 1:14).

They were in one accord in prayer, and the result shook the world! The Christians in the Early Church were in such unity that human selfishness seemed to almost disappear for a time. People shared their possessions and had all things in common. What power they had in prayer!

When violent persecution came, the record says, "They raised their voice to God with one accord ... And when they had prayed, the place where they were assembled together was shaken; and they were all filled with the Holy Spirit, and they spoke the word of God with boldness" (Acts 4:24,31). Instead of abating, the revival received fresh impetus and miracles of healing took place on a scale that amazed the nation.

UNITED PRAYER OPENED THE PRISON

Perhaps the most dramatic illustration of the power of united intercession is recorded in Acts 12. Persecution had reached the zenith of intensity. King Herod had killed James, the brother of John, with the sword. Then Peter was taken into custody, and was awaiting a similar fate.

But in the meantime, a company of prayer warriors gathered in the home of Mark's mother to continually intercede for the apostle. "Peter was therefore kept in prison, but constant prayer was offered to God for him by the church" (Acts 12:5).

The faith of this company was probably not at its highest peak. The startling news of the murder of one of the apostles had no doubt shaken them. It is unlikely that any one of them alone had the faith needed for a miracle of deliverance at that moment. This is evidenced by the fact that when Peter, after escaping from prison, came to their door and tried to enter, nobody believed it was actually he. If someone was there who looked like him, it must be his angel! Yet, in spite of the lack of faith, their united prayer touched heaven. Their combined faith, reached an intensity beyond what any one of them possessed.

Their prayer resulted in Herod's plan being completely frustrated. An angel opened the prison gates and led the apostle to safety. This is an example of how united prayer can meet any serious crisis that the Church may face.

The power of unity is nowhere more forcibly revealed than in Jesus' prayer that His disciples would become one. He was going to give the Church the solemn task of evangelizing the world. They were to tell everyone that He was the Christ Whom the Father had sent into the world. But how could the world be convinced that He was the Son of God?

The world would believe if: The Church presented a united front; the individual members were willing to subordinate their own plans and ambitions for the good of the whole; they would show the world they truly loved one another; and they would pray together in perfect agreement. "By this all will know that you are My disciples, if you have love for one another" (Jn. 13:35).

Jesus knew that if the disciples could bury their own personal ambitions so the believers would indeed become one, then the world would believe that He was the Christ. "That they all may be one, as You, Father, are in Me, and I in You; that they also may be one in Us, that the world may believe that You sent Me" (Jn. 17:21).

If two can put ten thousand to flight, how much would be accomplished if all of God's people became one? It would not be long until their united efforts would evangelize the world. If the

Christians from all nations would begin to pray fervently, many of their great problems would soon be solved!

HOW UNITED PRAYER SAVED A NATION

On May 10, 1940, the Nazi blitzkrieg was launched against the low countries. At the end of the second week in May, the French defenses at Sedan and on the Meuse were out, and the Nazi Panzers advanced openly through Belgium and France.

On Monday, May 29, the only port left to the British was Dunkirk. It looked as if Britain was about to face the most awful defeat in her history. The German High Command stated, "The British Army is encircled, our troops are proceeding to its annihilation."

The British government and people hoped only to gain time and start afresh. They did not expect to save more than 20-30 units, at the most, out of the debacle. A day of prayer had been called by His Majesty the King on May 26th; and God came to the defense of His people, controlling the weather! He caused a storm to descend in the area of Dunkirk, which saved the weary tramping armies from Nazi planes. Then He calmed the sea; it was so calm, the coastal yachts were used to transport troops from the beaches.

The next day, *The Daily Sketch* declared, "Nothing like it ever happened before." Everywhere, the word "miracle" was spoken. Soldiers and civilians alike, made mention of the *day of prayer*. The two strange weather conditions — the storm and the great calm —enabled the forces to save ten times the number even the most optimistic had hoped would be saved. Even large contingents of allied personnel were saved from the area.

Perhaps no one individual in England had faith for this miracle. In the natural, there was no hope. It seemed that within a few days, hundreds of thousands of English boys would either be dead or suffering in Nazi prison camps. But there were Christians praying in England, and a king who believed in prayer and had faith to call the nation to prayer in their hour of distress. God answered and the nation was saved.

WHEN JESUS ASKED HIS DISCIPLES TO HELP HIM PRAY

The power of united prayer is revealed by Jesus' words to His disciples on the night in Gethsemane. One might think Christ didn't need assistance in prayer. Surely He so thoroughly knew the art of praying that help from another person was not necessary. Yet when Jesus was agonizing in the garden, He asked His disciples to watch in prayer with Him. When He found they had fallen asleep, He said reproachfully, "What, could you not watch with Me one hour? Watch and pray, lest you enter into temptation. The spirit indeed is willing, but the flesh is weak" (Matt. 26:40,41).

Christ's statement to the disciples regarding their failure to watch with Him is a striking testimony of the power of united prayer. As great as Christ's power was in prayer, the prayers of others would have given Him hope in that difficult hour.

Agreeing in prayer is the biblical way of dealing with problems within the Church. By agreeing in prayer, the powers of hell can be bound and their evil schemes can be defeated. Jesus said:

> Assuredly, I say to you, whatever you bind on earth will be bound in heaven, and whatever you loose on earth will be loosed in heaven. Again I say to you that if two of you agree on earth concerning anything that they ask, it will be done for them by My Father in heaven (Matt. 18:18,19).

Another great secret of prayer is: One shall chase a thousand but two shall put ten thousand to flight. There is power in agreement. When special problems present themselves, choose a person who will agree with you for that particular thing. As you stand together in agreement, the answer will surely come. "Whatever you bind on earth will be bound in heaven, and whatever you loose on earth will be loosed in heaven."

CHAPTER XIII

The Secret By Which Power Can Be Increased 100-Fold

Likewise the Spirit also helps in our weaknesses. For we do not know what we should pray for as we ought, but the Spirit Himself makes intercession for us with groanings which cannot be uttered (Rom. 8:26).

Now we come to one of the greatest secrets of prayer. Just as a radio transmitting system can amplify the human voice so that it can reach over the whole world, so the power of the Spirit can amplify our feeble human efforts and make them powerful enough to move mountains.

In Genesis 1, we are told of the Spirit of God moving on the waters and bringing order out of the primeval chaos.

In the beginning God created the heavens and the earth. The earth was without form, and void; and darkness was on the face of the deep. And the Spirit of God was hovering over the face of the waters (Gen. 1:1,2).

When God's work was finished, the seas moved within their appointed bounds; the hills and mountains appeared in their proper places; the rivers flowed down the valleys into the seas, exactly as had been determined. But, it was not long before evil entered God's fair creation. So He had to restore His marred handiwork. He ordained prayer as the means of bringing His Spirit into the work of restoration.

The vital place the Spirit of God plays in answering prayer is clearly shown throughout the Scriptures. "It is the Spirit who gives life; the flesh profits nothing" (Jn. 6:63). The manner in which we allow the Spirit of God to move to our prayer life is of greatest importance.

The relation between praying and the moving of God's Spirit is clearly manifest in the life of Christ. In His first public act of baptism, as Christ came out of the water praying, the heavens opened and the Spirit of God descended on Him (Lk. 3:21,22). He was then led by the Spirit into the wilderness to spend 40 days in fasting and waiting upon God. There He met the devil face to face, and the sword of the Spirit successfully overcame all the temptations the prince of this world had to offer (Lk. 4:13).

Returning from the wilderness, Jesus called 12 disciples, and one of the first lessons He taught them was how to pray. The climax of His teaching was the great revelation that the Holy Spirit, Who previously had been reserved for a favored few, was now to be poured out on all flesh! Everyone who would ask the Heavenly Father would receive the Holy Spirit!

> And I say to you, ask, and it will be given to you; seek, and you will find; knock, and it will be opened to you. For everyone who asks receives, and he who seeks finds, and to him who knocks it will be opened. ... If you then, being evil, know how to give good gifts to your children, how much more will your heavenly Father give the Holy Spirit to those who ask Him! (Lk. 11:9,10,13).

SPIRITUAL WARFARE

In Ephesians 6:10-18, the apostle Paul speaks of spiritual warfare. He declares that a Christian does "not wrestle against flesh and blood, but against principalities, against powers, against the rulers of the darkness of this age, against spiritual hosts of wickedness in the heavenly places" (Eph. 6:12). After listing the spiritual armor necessary to stand against the enemy, Paul shows the Christian how to prosecute this warfare by praying in the Spirit.

> Praying always with all prayer and supplication in the
> Spirit, being watchful to this end with all perseverance
> and supplication for all the saints (Eph. 6:18).

The reason many people are not able to pray with power is because they have not learned to pray in the Spirit. They know they need additional power. They confess that they often meet opposition in prayer that is beyond their strength to overcome. What is the answer to their problem? The solution is learning to pray in the Spirit.

To successfully pray for a lost world, one needs the power of the Holy Spirit. To war against principalities and spiritual wickedness in high places, one needs the presence of the Spirit. To minister to the sick in body and soul, one needs the compassion of the Spirit. To exercise the gifts of the Spirit, one needs the quickening of the Spirit. A Christian only fails, if he attempts to do these things in his own strength.

Here is the secret we must learn: God hears the prayers of the weakest saint, but to pray with power — taking the spiritual offensive — it is necessary to pray in the Spirit. That is why Paul showed the great part the Spirit should have in our prayer life:

> Likewise the Spirit also helps in our weaknesses. For we
> do not know what we should pray for as we ought, but
> the Spirit Himself makes intercession for us with
> groanings which cannot be uttered (Rom. 8:26).

The believer needs the Holy Spirit's help in prayer. Often a person does not know what to pray for. He does not know what temptations lie ahead. The Spirit of God, however, knows if pitfalls lie ahead. He will, if given the opportunity, pray effectively against the danger. It is known that others need prayer, but it is the Spirit

Who knows *which* person has a critical need at a given time. All need wisdom in making decisions, especially those that must be made on short notice. The Spirit of God knows all, and if given opportunity, will prepare the believer for that decision. His omniscience and omnipotence will cause all things to work together for good. It is not coincidence that the two great truths of Romans 8:26 and 28 are revealed together — for one follows the other. *If* the Spirit of God prays through us, we can be sure He will cause everything to work out for good!

HOW DO WE PRAY IN THE SPIRIT?

Now we come to the important question: How does a person pray in the Spirit? How does the Spirit of God pray through him? The answer is simple. As long as he is praying in his own language, he is doing the praying. *But when praying in the unknown tongue, the Spirit of God does the praying.* Paul explains this in I Corinthians 14:14,15:

> For if I pray in an unknown tongue, my spirit prays, but
> my understanding is unfruitful. What is the result then?
> I will pray with the spirit, and I will also pray with the
> understanding.

There is praying with the Spirit and praying with the understanding. Paul prayed with the understanding and he also prayed with the Spirit — that is, in an unknown tongue. Though he spoke in the unknown tongue little in public, he prayed a great deal in the Spirit in private. In fact he could say, "I thank my God I speak with tongues more than you all" (I Cor. 14:18). He knew the importance of praying in the Spirit.

Without praying in the Spirit, it is possible to overlook things of vital importance. There may be opposition not anticipated. There may be unexpected problems. The Holy Spirit, however, is able to cope with every circumstance and problem. If a Christian's faith fails, he can, by the Spirit's praying through him, move into the orbit of God's faith. When the Spirit prays, the supernatural comes into operation, and the miracle comes to pass.

There are people who have prayed years for a certain thing, but their faith seemed never able to get the answer. Then suddenly, as the Spirit of God moved upon them in prayer, the miracle took place. So Zechariah 4:6 is fulfilled: "'Not by might nor by power, but by My Spirit,' says the LORD of hosts."

THE MIRACLE IN LONDON

In 1952, I had made plans to go to a world conference in London, England, where I was scheduled to speak. Then I intended to fulfill my life-long dream of visiting the Holy Land.

A day or two before I was to leave, I received distressing news: My mother had suddenly suffered a severe stroke which had affected her mind. So serious was the attack she was unable to recognize anyone.

A stroke affecting the brain is always grave, but at the age of 78 as she was, the result is usually fatal. Perhaps it was her time to go; but if so, I certainly wanted to be near her. In Israel, I would not have contact with home for several weeks. What should I do?

This situation placed me in an awkward position. Was it God's will that I cancel my trip to London and the Holy Land? I prayed, but it was difficult to arrive at a conclusion. However, my relatives felt that I should go, and so with some misgivings, I flew to England. Faith is action, and it was a step of faith to make this decision.

Arriving in London, I was restless in my spirit and spent considerable time in prayer in my room at the Baker Street Hotel. The seriousness of the attack and my mother's advanced age made me realize that nothing less than an unusual miracle would cause her to recover. The whole situation weighed heavily on me. I continued in prayer, but finally admitted to myself, I was getting nowhere.

As I knelt in my room, depressed and baffled by the circumstances, something seemed to say, "If this mountain is too great for you to move, why don't you let the Holy Spirit move it?" The force of these words impressed me greatly. I continued to kneel, but did not pray. For perhaps half an hour I remained motionless, not saying a word. Then the Spirit began to move. I began to pray in an unknown tongue; but it was not I praying, it was the Spirit within me. Prayer began to roll in a torrent. The Spirit of God was rebuking death! He was abolishing sickness! There was not the slightest doubt that things were happening now. How long I continued in prayer I do not know. But suddenly I found myself on my feet, and on my way back to the convention hall. All my anxiety was gone, and there was no doubt in my mind that God had taken care of the situation.

From London I went to the Holy Land. Several weeks later, I returned to Paris where my wife's niece was preparing to go to Africa as a missionary. She handed me a letter from my mother. She wrote praises to God for her complete deliverance! I was not surprised. I knew that a miracle took place that day while I was in my room in London. Where I failed, the Spirit of God brought the answer.

It is possible for the Spirit to move on one's praying until it seems God becomes completely identified with the individual who is praying. Such experiences come only to those who learn to wait upon the Lord. "But those who wait on the LORD shall renew their strength; they shall mount up with wings like eagles, they shall run and not be weary, they shall walk and not faint" (Isa. 40:31).

Those who wait on the Lord renew their strength. Many want to rush into the presence of the Lord. They do not take time to still their minds before Him. They are so active, they never give opportunity for the Spirit to enter into their praying.

David knew what it was to wait on God. He declared: "Rest in the LORD, and wait patiently for Him ... For evildoers shall be cut off; But those who wait on the LORD, they shall inherit the earth" (Psa. 37:7,9).

Not only will mountains be given into our hands, but the whole earth! By waiting on God, David won mighty victories, sometimes against great odds. He learned to take counsel from the Lord before each move. Once, the Philistines were coming against him. Should he go out to meet them? God said, "Not yet." He was to wait until he heard "the sound of marching in the tops of the mulberry trees, then you shall advance quickly. For then the LORD will go out before you ..." (II Sam. 5:24). David was to wait until the Spirit moved; then he would know the time for victory had come.

After they witnessed Christ's resurrection, the apostles were ready to go and witness. But Jesus said, "Not yet. Wait for the promise of the Father." Obeying, they returned to the upper room where they "continued with one accord in prayer and supplication" (Acts 1:14). On the day of Pentecost, suddenly there was a breath from heaven. That breath became a mighty rushing wind. The Spirit of God fell upon the disciples in such power, a revival began that shook the world.

Here is another great secret in the art of prayer. If it seems you are making slow progress, if your prayers do not appear to be getting through or if a wall of resistance confronts you, wait upon the Lord. Learn to let the Spirit move. Wait, as David did, for the "marching in the tops of the mulberry trees." When the Spirit moves, give Him full permission; let Him pray through you. He will succeed where you would fail. He knows how to pray, what to pray for and how to get the answer. He will enable your power in prayer to be increased 100-fold!

CHAPTER XIV

The Secret of the Unseen Enemy

For we do not wrestle against flesh and blood, but against principalities, against powers, against the rulers of the darkness of this age, against spiritual hosts of wickedness in the heavenly places (Eph. 6:12).

Prayer is spiritual warfare. Unseen spiritual powers are real and arrayed against believers. Without a vigorous prayer life, a believer is at the mercy of these unseen powers. Prayerless people are driven by sinister forces of which they are usually unaware. Few Christians recognize the extent evil powers can exert in their affairs. People concern themselves mainly with flesh and blood, using their strength to battle against opposition they can see. They do not realize that flesh and blood are not the real enemy.

Paul reveals the nature of the Christian's warfare. The wrestling is not against flesh and blood, but against rulers of the darkness of this world. In Ephesians 6:13-18, he designates the armor and the weapons that we need to make a successful warfare. (It would be good for the reader to carefully read these verses.)

PRAYER — A WAR AGAINST THE DEVIL!

Equipped with this armor, the Christian is to offensively pray against the devil. "Praying always with all prayer and supplication in the Spirit, being watchful to this end with all perseverance and supplication for all the saints" (Eph. 6:18). Spiritual warfare is against a real enemy; one who seeks to take advantage of any opening.

In the days of Job, when the sons of God came to present themselves before the Lord, "Satan also came among them" (Job 1:6). The devil showed up too, with the purpose of causing trouble. For reasons I cannot take the time to go into here, God allowed Satan to attack Job for a season. Satan did his worst. He directed the Sabeans to attack Job's servants. He caused lightning to strike Job's herds and consume them. He was the author of the cyclone which destroyed the building where Job's children were. It was the devil who put painful boils on Job (Job 2:7). Job said, "The LORD gave, and the LORD has taken away" (Job 1:21). It *was* God who gave; but it was the devil who took away!

What startling things could be seen if a person's senses were able to discern what really takes place in the heavenlies. The Bible gives us a view of what transpires in the spirit world.

THE "PRINCE OF PERSIA"

In Daniel 10, we see a glimpse of the devil's activities on a worldwide scale. Here, one of Satan's chief lieutenants is described as the "prince of Persia." Every nation has a prince of the kingdom of darkness assigned to it. This powerful spirit prince has a legion of lesser spirits under him. They carry out his orders, and through them, Satan maintains his kingdom and accomplishes his purpose of seducing and deceiving men.

At the time of Daniel's prayer, three years had passed since the first company of Jews had returned to Jerusalem through a gracious answer to prayer. Yet Daniel knew that not all was going well. The constant harassment the Jews suffered in their native land spelled trouble for the future. Daniel wondered what would happen to his nation in future generations. The afflictions of his people weighed heavy on his heart. He wanted to know what would happen to them in centuries to come. He was so burdened about the matter, he set aside time to meditate and seek God, asking that He would reveal these things to him.

Daniel was used to getting his prayers answered. When at first, he received no answer, the prophet was not discouraged. Instead he was spurred on to new efforts. It was his rule never to give up until the answer came. He gave himself to prayer and fasting. Days passed with no indication that God heard him. Three weeks went by and still no answer.

Then on the twenty-first day, something happened! An angel from God suddenly entered his room! According to the angel, Daniel's petition had been heard the very first day, and God had immediately sent him to bring the answer. But an evil power, "the prince of Persia" had hindered him. The angel said:

> Do not fear, Daniel, for from the first day that you set your heart to understand, and to humble yourself before your God, your words were heard; and I have come because of your words. But the prince of the kingdom of Persia withstood me twenty-one days; and behold, Michael, one of the chief princes, came to help me, for I had been left alone there with the kings of Persia (Dan. 10:12,13).

This is perhaps one of the most remarkable revelations in the Old Testament. These verses give a unique glimpse into what takes place in the unseen world. The "prince of Persia" was not like a human ruler, who would not have power to resist an angel. He was a spirit prince under Satan. The unseen powers of darkness inhabit the heavenlies, and manipulate events in the world (of course, within the limits of divine permission).

There is a spiritual kingdom composed of principalities and powers. Every nation on earth has an unseen spirit ruler. Earthly kingdoms are under the influence of organized forces of wickedness which seek to bend them completely to their will.

Then the devil, taking Him up on a high mountain, showed Him all the kingdoms of the world in a moment of time. And the devil said to Him, "All this authority I will give You, and their glory; for this has been delivered to me, and I give it to whomever I wish" (Lk. 4:5,6).

Under Satan, there are subordinate princes, who in turn, have armies of demons under them. They work toward one purpose — to bring all inhabitants of this planet under their control. Those who suppose man evolved from a lower species and will become a super-race that can create its own millennium are under great delusion. Human attempts at race regeneration are hopelessly impotent. Only the power of the Gospel can have any effect in changing man's fallen nature.

Spiritual powers in high places can be dislodged only by spiritual warfare. The "prince of Persia" is strong: For three weeks he was able to successfully hinder the angel from getting through to Daniel. He highly resented his authority being disturbed, and fiercely resisted intrusion into his domain. Nevertheless, Daniel continued praying, and when God sent reinforcements by the Archangel Michael the powers of darkness were at last forced to give way.

What if Daniel had given up? The answer is unmistakable. Daniel's faithfulness in prayer had a determining effect on the outcome of the struggle in the heavenlies. Because he persisted in prayer, the "prince of Persia" was defeated.

FINNEY, THE MAN WHO PRAYED DOWN REVIVALS

A memorable example of the believer's conflict with principalities and powers, occurred when Charles G. Finney interceded for revival. He was on board a ship returning home from Europe. For 12-14 years, he had been engaged in a series of revival meetings that had influenced America as no other had. But overwork had strained his health, and he had taken a trip to restore his strength. While he was resting, news came of anti-slavery agitation. He was filled with anxiety over whether this confusion would hinder revival. He tells about how the spirit of prayer was upon him, enabling him to prevail with God:

> On my homeward passage, my mind became exceedingly exercised on the question of revivals. I feared that they would decline throughout the country. My own health, it appeared to me, had nearly or quite broken down; and I knew of no other evangelist that would take the field, and aid the pastors in the revival work. This view of the subject distressed me so much that one day I found myself unable to rest. My soul was in an utter agony. I spent almost the entire day in prayer in my stateroom, or walking the deck in intense agony, in view of the state of things. In fact, I felt crushed with the burden that was on my soul. There was no one aboard to whom I could open my mind, or say a word.

> It was the spirit of prayer that was upon me; that which I had often before experienced, but perhaps never before to such a degree, for so long a time. I besought the Lord to go on with His work and to provide Himself with such instrumentalities as were necessary. After a day of unspeakable wrestling and agony in my soul, just at night, the subject cleared up in my mind. The Spirit led me to believe that all would come out right and that God had yet a work for me to do; that I might be at rest; that the Lord would go forward with His work.

Why was it necessary for Finney to wrestle so long in prayer? Why couldn't the Lord give him the answer at once? Because first a battle had to be won in the heavenlies. Satan opposed the great revival. It was the crucial hour. If the devil could have discouraged Finney before the spiritual battle had been won, the revival could have been stopped. But because he, like Daniel, would not be denied — wrestling until God sent reinforcements — the great revival continued.

This great visitation under Finney's leadership reached a climax in 1857-58, when an unprecedented revival prevailed throughout the northern states. Finney says, "It swept over the land with such power, that for a time it was estimated that not less than fifty thousand conversions occurred in a single week. Indeed, daily prayer meetings were established through the length and breadth of the Northern states."

If revival had spread to the south, perhaps the Civil War could have been averted. Apparently there was no man in the south who could wrestle in prayer as Finney did. The need for someone to intercede until the answer comes is seen in Ezekiel 22:30-31:

> So I sought for a man among them who would make a wall, and stand in the gap before Me on behalf of the land, that I should not destroy it; but I found no one. Therefore I have poured out My indignation on them; I have consumed them with the fire of My wrath.

You and I do not wrestle against flesh and blood, but against principalities and powers in high places. Spiritual "mountains" — kingdoms, as it were — oppose us. But if a person stays steady in prayer, God will send the necessary reinforcements for victory. Never accept failure or defeat. Though the answer be delayed, it will surely come. To move mountains, you must not allow yourself to be moved.

CHAPTER XV

The Secret of the Authority of Prayer

And whatever you ask in My name, that I will do, that
the Father may be glorified in the Son (Jn. 14:13).

Unlimited power is available to those who pray. By faith, the
believer can move the mountain standing in his way. The inevitable
question is: By whose authority can one speak to the mountain and
say, "Be removed"? By whose authority can we speak to the
elements and demand that they obey us?

The universe is governed by law and order. So are the angels of
heaven. Even demons recognize and respect God's authority. The
pharisees knew that miracles must be performed through authority.
When they saw the mighty works of Jesus, they were puzzled. By
what power did He do these things? They decided they must find
out.

THE AUTHORITY OF JESUS

The same day Jesus spoke about the power of faith (Matt.
21:21,22), the pharisees came to question Him. Apparently He was
discussing this subject when the pharisees listened in. So Jesus was
talking about moving mountains, was He? Well, who gave Him
authority to say and do all these things? They turned to Jesus and
said, "By what authority are You doing these things? And who gave
You this authority?" (Matt. 21:23).

The haughty pharisees did not get much satisfaction from Jesus' answer. Refusing to gratify their curiosity, He asked a counter-question, which they saw would embarrass them to answer. They left more frustrated and angry than ever.

But Christ had already revealed the secret of His authority. He had told the Jews before, that He had come in His Father's name (Jn. 5:43). He did the miracles because His Father gave Him the authority. He raised the dead because His Father had given Him the power (Jn. 5:21,28,29). It was no secret where Jesus got His authority. It was given Him by His Father.

THE AUTHORITY OF THE BELIEVER

Now we come to a parallel question. Jesus' power came from His Father, but where does the believer's come from? Does he get it directly from the Father as Jesus did? No, he does not. No man is worthy to approach the Father as Jesus approached Him. All who come to the Father must come through Jesus. "I am the way, the truth, and the life. No one comes to the Father except through Me" (Jn. 14:6). The power to deliver, heal the sick and to set the bound free comes through Christ.

This is the secret of New Testament prayer and the believer's authority. All that the Christian has, comes through Christ. There is no salvation, healing, deliverance or power over Satan, except through the name of Jesus, and through the authority of His name.

When Jesus had risen from the dead and ascended to the Father, the disciples began to do the mighty works Jesus had commanded them to do. The pharisees heard what was happening, and came to Peter and John just after they had healed the lame man at the gate Beautiful. Amazed by what they saw, they demanded, "By what power or by what name have you done this?" (Acts 4:7). Peter responded to their questions by saying:

> Let it be known to you all, and to all the people of Israel,
> that by the name of Jesus Christ of Nazareth, whom you
> crucified, whom God raised from the dead, by Him this

man stands here before you whole. ... Nor is there salvation in any other, for there is no other name under heaven given among men by which we must be saved (Acts 4:10,12).

THE POWER OF ATTORNEY

Jesus, in giving the use of His Name to His followers, gave them the power of attorney. That is, He gave them His authority to use. When they used His power, it would be the same as if He used it. "As the Father has sent Me, I also send you" (Jn. 20:21). In the same manner Christ received authority from the Father, He passed it on to His followers.

In giving the disciples the use of His Name, Jesus gave them unlimited power. All power in heaven and in earth has been delivered to Christ; therefore, all power in heaven and in earth has also been given to His disciples.

The reason many Christians have so little power in their lives is not because the power is not available, but because they fail to use it. Suppose a millionaire who has unlimited funds in a bank gave you a checkbook with his name signed at the bottom of each check and said, "Use whatever you wish." Would it do you any good if you didn't fill out one of the checks and go to the bank and cash it? Great power has been given to you, but it will not do you any good unless you fill out the checks and present them to the bank of heaven to honor.

It is perhaps beyond human comprehension why Christ would entrust His followers with such great power. But it is true. Unlimited power is at the believer's command; not for personal power or position, not for ease and gratification; but to bring the blessing of heaven upon suffering humanity. Any other use would be an abuse of the power granted.

THE POWER OF THE NAME OF JESUS

Some years ago in an evangelistic meeting we directed, an incident happened which proved before several thousand people the power of the name of Jesus. The evangelist told the audience, that if they would believe the song they had just sung — *Only believe, all things are possible, only believe* — they would see mighty miracles that night. As he was saying this, we noticed a man rapidly advancing up the aisle toward the platform.

As he came closer, we were startled by his demonic countenance. At first we thought somebody had brought an insane man to the service and that he had broken loose and was now coming up the platform to make a disturbance. Later we learned that he was not insane, but a vicious character who had previously entered area churches and created serious disturbances. He had been arrested, but jail sentences had not taught him a lesson. Now he had seized this opportunity to create another commotion.

By the time he reached the platform, the congregation had noticed his menacing attitude. As we were calling the evangelist's attention to what was taking place, two strong police officers came rushing out of the wings. They had seen what was happening and were about to wrestle the disturber. They could have done so, but it probably would have ruined the service, so the evangelist waved them back.

After asking the audience to bow their heads in prayer, he walked over to where the man stood. As he did so, the antagonist began to curse him saying, "You are of the devil and deceiving the people, an impostor, a snake in the grass, and I am going to show the people that you are." It was a bold challenge and everyone could see it was not an idle threat. As the intruder continued his abuse, mingled with hissing and spitting, he lifted his hands as if to follow through with his threats. The officers made another move to come to the evangelist's aid, but again they were waved away.

Critics in the auditorium out of curiosity that night no doubt expected a swift and pitiful conclusion to this unscheduled drama. In this moment of suspense we were reminded of Goliath's challenge when he cursed David in the name of his gods, then boasted he would tear him limb from limb.

Seconds passed, but the intruder was not proceeding with his boasts of physical violence. Something was hindering the challenger from carrying out his evil intent. Softly but determinedly, the evangelist said, "Satan, because you have challenged the servant of God before this audience, you must, in the name of Jesus, fall at my feet!" As the mighty name of Jesus was spoken, we could see something happening! The strong forces controlling the evil challenger were submitting to the power of the name of Jesus! Suddenly, the man who had so brazenly defied the man of God with threats and accusations, gave an awful groan and slumped to the floor sobbing hysterically.

It was the name of Jesus which brought the result! No other name in heaven and earth has the power of the name of Jesus. It is greater than any other name. That name is your authority. By that name all things are yours. Jesus said, "If you ask anything in My name, I will do it" (Jn. 14:14).

Using the name of Jesus only has results for true believers. Those who are disobedient to God's will have no right to use it, nor will demons respond when they do so. Demons know the difference between a real Christian and a phony.

Jewish vagabonds, who dabbled in spiritism, thought that the name of Jesus would work like a magic charm. They tried to exorcise evil spirits by this name of Jesus, saying, "We adjure you by the Jesus whom Paul preaches" (Acts 19:13). The evil spirits responded by saying, "Jesus I know, and Paul I know; but who are you?" (Acts 19:15). The man who had the evil spirit overpowered them and they ran in terror, naked and wounded.

The secret of the believer's authority in prayer is in the name of Jesus. As the Father has committed all power to the Son, so the Son commits all power to those who trust in Him. It is the power of His name — the power of His authority. Christ repeats the promise over and over. Whatever believers ask in His name, He will do (Jn. 14:13). If they ask anything in His name, He will do it (Jn. 14:14). They are to ask in His Name and receive, that their joy may be full (Jn. 16:24). They are to cast out devils and heal the sick in His name (Mk. 16:17,18). All things are possible — even moving mountains — if God's people ask in the name of Jesus.

CHAPTER XVI

The Secret of the Faith that Moves Mountains

So Jesus answered and said to them, "Have faith in God. For assuredly, I say to you, whoever says to this mountain, 'Be removed and be cast into the sea,' and does not doubt in his heart, but believes that those things he says will come to pass, he will have whatever he says. Therefore I say to you, whatever things you ask when you pray, believe that you receive them, and you will have them" (Mk. 11:22-24).

These startling words were spoken by Jesus when He was standing on an actual mountain — the Mount of Olives. The previous day, He had journeyed over the mountain from Bethany. He had seen a fig tree in the distance, and stopped to eat some. To His disappointment, He found the tree had nothing but leaves. Then He spoke to the fig tree, "Let no one eat fruit from you ever again" (Mk. 11:14).

The disciples heard what He said. They looked at the tree, but saw no immediate change. The foliage was still as green as ever. But the following day, as they passed by again, they were startled to see the leaves had withered away. Peter called attention to this and said, "Rabbi, look! The fig tree which You cursed has withered away" (Mk. 11:21). This remark of Peter's, brought Christ's amazing statement of the power of faith.

What happened to the fig tree when it was cursed? Actually, at the very moment Jesus spoke the word, the fig tree died. But it took time for the results to be manifested. In this remarkable incident, Jesus revealed another vital secret of prayer: Believing must precede receiving. "Whatever things you ask when you pray, believe that you receive them, and you will have them" (Mk. 11:24). We are not to believe we will receive at a future time. That would be denying that God has already answered prayer, that He has kept His Word. We must believe it happens at the moment we ask, though there may not be the slightest evidence of change. Jesus taught that the answer comes the moment a believer prays in faith — even though it is yet invisible to the natural eye.

Jesus praised God for the raising of Lazarus while he was still in the tomb. The believer is to believe he has the answer simply because God's Word says so. What can be seen or felt with the senses has nothing to do with it. To those who believe, the invisible must become visible and the visible become invisible.

Blessing are not received because they are deserved or have been prayed for, or because of some desperate need. Faith never looks at conditions or symptoms. Faith disregards what the natural senses discern. Faith created the world when there was nothing. Faith is only faith when it sees nothing. Once the answer comes it is no longer faith, but sight. Faith rests completely upon the Word of God. "Whatever things you ask when you pray, believe that you receive them, and you will have them" (Mk. 11:24).

MUSTARD-SEED FAITH

Faith to move mountains! Most people think that kind of faith is unattainable. Yet this faith is not something extraordinary. It is simply a persistent and sustained faith — one that does not weaken under testing. It is a faith that rejects the natural senses and regards God's Word as the supreme determining factor of whether a thing is true. This is mustard-seed faith, which Jesus said was all that was necessary to move mountains.

> If you have faith as a mustard seed, you will say to this mountain, "Move from here to there," and it will move; and nothing will be impossible for you (Matt. 17:20).

There is nothing spectacular about a mustard seed. Plant it in the ground, and if it is dug up the next day, there is no change in its appearance. Look at it a week later and there may still be little change. But something has been set in motion. Billions of little atoms are at work rearranging themselves in creating the first cells of a mustard tree. Down in the dark soil, microscopically small movement has begun.

While the change is exceedingly slow, it is incessant. Days pass, and finally a tiny plant breaks through the soil. Higher and higher the little plant shoots up. That growth doesn't stop until the will of God for the development of a mustard tree is fulfilled — until birds are able to find lodging in its branches. Mustard-seed faith is not a spectacular faith, but it is an unrelenting faith. That is the faith Jesus said will move the mountains.

Why do mountains sometimes fail to move? The reason usually is not difficult to find. Most people plant their mustard seed, and then dig it up again. They mistake mustard-seed faith for instantaneous faith. They plant the seed, but return shortly to examine it. When the change cannot be seen, they think nothing has happened. They say, "I am still sick! My symptoms are still here! I didn't get my healing!" By confessing failure they uproot the seed of their faith. They accept defeat, when victory was already on the way. The seed began to grow the moment they planted it, but their faith wavers. They think mustard-seed faith not only moves mountains, but that it happens overnight. When that doesn't happen, they give in to failure.

HE BELIEVED GOD AND 400,000 PEOPLE ATTENDED ONE SERVICE

Some years ago we received a letter from Evangelist Tommy Hicks informing us he was going to Argentina to hold a revival. He said he had prayed a long time about the matter, and now the time had come for him to go. He added that he knew God was going to give him a great harvest in that country.

Argentina was not an easy field at that time. The nation was held in the grip of a strong dictatorship. Actually, the evangelist didn't know who was president of Argentina. But when he arrived in Lima, Peru, God spoke the name "Peron" to him while he was in prayer. He inquired at the airline office, and was informed that Peron was the president of Argentina. There was no doubt in his mind that God wanted him to speak to this man personally.

When Hicks arrived in Buenos Aires, he made his purpose known. He was told the plan could never succeed. The proposal seemed absurd. Peron was always surrounded with guards and secret agents, and ordinarily, only those with important official business were permitted an appointment.

Nevertheless, Tommy Hicks believed that God would open the way. He decided to make an attempt to see Peron. Arriving at the palace, he requested an interview with the president. Somehow God arranged a meeting. Hicks obtained favor from the president. Peron allowed himself to be photographed with Hicks after the interview. He granted Hicks the unheard of privilege of holding revival meetings in the largest stadiums in the country. And before Hicks left Peron, he was permitted to pray with him.

A campaign that made history began. Crowds reached 100,000 and they had to move to one seating 200,000. Soon that stadium, too was filled. Before the campaign was over, it is said the same number of people were on the outside clamoring to get in. And so the nation of Argentina was shaken as a result of the prayers and faith of the people of God.

CAN REAL MOUNTAINS BE MOVED?

When Jesus spoke of moving mountains, did He mean real mountains? As we have already seen, the expression "mountain" has figurative application. A "mountain" may signify any powerful opposition that stands in the way of our progress. But the promise of moving mountains includes real mountains — although it may be rare that a literal mountain needs to be moved.

Note that Jesus spoke of *"this mountain"* in Mark 11:23. "This mountain" on which He was standing actually the Mount of Olives, located just east of Jerusalem (Mk. 11:11,12). Prophecy declares that the Mount of Olives will someday be moved from its present location! During the great day of the Lord when judgment will fall on the nations that have come up against Jerusalem, Christ will again stand on the Mount of Olives — perhaps near the spot where He cursed the fig tree. The Mount of Olives will split in the center — half toward the south, and half toward the north — and the waters shall flow through where the Mount of Olives once stood:

> And in that day His feet will stand on the Mount of Olives, which faces Jerusalem on the east. And the Mount of Olives shall be split in two, from east to west, making a very large valley; half of the mountain shall move toward the north and half of it toward the south. ... And in that day it shall be that living waters shall flow from Jerusalem, half of them toward the eastern sea and half of them toward the western sea; in both summer and winter it shall occur (Zech. 14:4,8).

God has a time for moving the mountains! In the Book of Revelation at the opening of the fifth seal, the martyred saints are petitioning God to "avenge our blood on those who dwell on the earth" (Rev. 6:10). They inquire of the Lord how long they must wait. They are told to rest a little while longer, until the others who are yet to be martyred fulfill their course. But God does not forget their prayers. Being gracious, He delays so everyone will have a chance to repent. Yet the hour must come when mercy ends. The trumpet angels begin to sound as they offer up "the prayers of all the saints upon the golden altar which was before the throne" (Rev. 8:3). Note what follows:

> Then the second angel sounded: And something like a great mountain burning with fire was thrown into the sea,

and a third of the sea became blood; and a third of the living creatures in the sea died, and a third of the ships were destroyed (Rev. 8:8,9).

WHEN THE SUN AND THE MOON STOOD STILL

Praying in the will of God has changed things greater than mountains. In the days of Joshua, the children of Israel were engaged in deadly combat against the people of Canaan. They had won a great victory, but night was coming. In the dark, their enemies, familiar with the land, would flee to the mountains. Then the Israelites might not be able to conquer them again. Joshua commanded the sun and the moon to stand still in their orbit. And they obeyed his command!

> Then Joshua spoke to the LORD ... in the sight of Israel: "Sun, stand still over Gibeon; and Moon, in the Valley of Aijalon." So the sun stood still, and the moon stopped, till the people had revenge upon their enemies. Is this not written in the Book of Jasher? So the sun stood still in the midst of heaven, and did not hasten to go down for about a whole day (Josh. 10:12,13).

Just stopping the sun was certainly a tremendous miracle. But consider Isaiah, who as the result of Hezekiah's prayer, caused the sun to go backward ten degrees on the dial of Ahaz (Isa. 38:8)!

The secret of prayer that moves mountains is faith based upon the Word of God and the will of God. All that is required is mustard-seed faith, which never relents until the answer is complete. The fulfillment of the promise does not depend on sight or feelings, only upon God's Word. "Whatever things you ask when you pray, believe that you receive them, and you will have them" (Mk. 11:24).

CHAPTER XVII

The Secret of Prayer and Fasting

For assuredly, I say to you, if you have faith as a mustard seed, you will say to this mountain, "Move from here to there," and it will move; and nothing will be impossible for you. However, this kind does not go out except by prayer and fasting (Matt. 17:20,21).

Jesus had just performed a startling miracle. An epileptic boy had been brought to the disciples for healing. They had tried to cast out the demon, but had failed. Perhaps some thought that since the apostles could not heal the boy, it was the will of God for him to remain that way. But Jesus quickly healed the child. He explained that the disciples had been unable to heal the lad because of their unbelief.

He said that if the disciples had faith as a grain of mustard seed, they could say to the mountain, "Be removed," and it would obey. That was the power of faith. But the question was, how could they get such faith? *Jesus answered this question by disclosing another vital secret in the art of praying.* He said, "However, this kind does not go out except by prayer and fasting" (Matt. 17:21).

Jesus was saying that certain evil spirits are so powerful, that prayer and fasting are necessary to overcome them. Demons, such as the one in the epileptic boy, could not be dislodged except through fasting. There are certain rules that must be adhered to if one's fasting is to be effective. When Jesus gave His lesson on prayer in Matthew 6, He also spoke of fasting. He showed some of the mistakes that are made in fasting. Even in a humble act such as fasting, human pride can enter. Some fast just to receive honor of men. This is vain and without profit. Jesus said,

> Moreover, when you fast, do not be like the hypocrites, with a sad countenance. For they disfigure their faces that they may appear to men to be fasting. Assuredly, I say to you, they have their reward. But you, when you fast, anoint your head and wash your face, so that you do not appear to men to be fasting, but to your Father who is in the secret place; and your Father who sees in secret will reward you openly (Matt. 6:16-18).

We need to learn the right way to fast. Some fast for aesthetic or health reasons. Others fast to have God's power in their lives. But some fast for strife:

> Indeed you fast for strife and debate, and to strike with the fist of wickedness. You will not fast as you do this day, to make your voice heard on high. Is it a fast that I have chosen, a day for a man to afflict his soul? ... Would you call this a fast, and an acceptable day to the LORD? Is this not the fast that I have chosen: to loose the bonds of wickedness, to undo the heavy burdens, to let the oppressed go free, and that you break every yoke? (Isa. 58:4-6).

Fasting is not a matter for strife and debate. Fasting is to assist us in bringing God's deliverance to those that are bound. Fasting is to draw us out of the natural and into the spiritual. Fasting is to quicken the faculties. Fasting is a means of implementing and strengthening prayer. Fasting and praying make faith strong enough to cast out demons.

HOW LONG SHOULD A PERSON FAST?

How long should a person fast? Ordinary fasts last only a short time. Cornelius fasted until three o'clock in the afternoon. Paul fasted three days as recorded in Acts 9:9. Short and frequent fasts should be a norm in the Christian life (I Cor. 7:5; Mk. 2:18-20; II Cor. 11:27).

Long fasts are also recorded in Scripture. Most of these were because of some overwhelming need. For instance, Moses fasted forty days when it appeared that Israel was about to perish under divine judgment (Ex. 32:10; 34:28).

There were times when Daniel fasted for long periods. Once when a prince of Satan withstood the answer to his prayer — that God intended to be answered the first day — Daniel, "ate no pleasant food" for three weeks. Ultimately the answer came (Dan. 10:2,3,12).

Christ began His ministry after He had fasted forty days. He was "filled with the Holy Spirit" (Lk. 4:1) before He fasted, but afterward, "He returned in the power of the Spirit" (Lk. 4:14).

Fasting is the answer when a mountain must be moved. Sometimes people find themselves in a place of hopelessness from which they cannot extricate themselves. Others are so oppressed by Satan, they cannot get free. There are circumstances where innocent become the victim of the foolishness of others. Is there hope for these? Fasting is the answer in these cases.

Paul was a prisoner on board a ship moving toward disaster. A violent wind tossed the ship for days until it seemed there was no hope. Paul, having been forewarned of God, had begged the captain not to make the journey, but his advice had not been heeded. Trouble often comes as a result of people failing to heed the revealed will of God. During those dark days when all hope seemed gone, Paul and the seamen fasted. God heard Paul's prayer and promised that all on board, for his sake, would be saved (Acts 27:33,34).

When other means fail, fasting is the answer. When efforts to cast out a stubborn demon are unsuccessful, it is time to fast. When every attempt to move the mountain that stands in the way of victory fails, then it is time for fasting.

When all other means fail, God has given us the resource of fasting. Prayer and fasting must eventually move the mountain that is standing in the way.

Here is another great secret of prayer. If there is a mountain standing in the way — an especially hard case, an affliction that refuses to budge, a demon that refuses to be exorcised — then prayer and fasting is the answer. Mountains must crumble before those who pray and fast. For them nothing shall be impossible!

CHAPTER XVIII

The Secret of Dominion in Prayer

Assuredly, I say to you, if you have faith and do not doubt, you will not only do what was done to the fig tree, but also if you say to this mountain, "Be removed and be cast into the sea," it will be done. And all things, whatever you ask in prayer, believing, you will receive (Matt. 21:21,22).

The above verses call attention to a little-recognized element in the art of prayer. Effective prayer must have the spirit of dominion. Having prayed the prayer of faith, we must be ready to command in faith. One of the purposes of prayer is to prepare us to take dominion over the elements and bend them to the will of God.

This is in harmony with the original purpose of God when He said, "Let Us make man in Our image, according to Our likeness; let them have dominion ... over all the earth" (Gen. 1:26). Man was not to be beaten by the elements; he was to conquer, control and bring them into subjection to the divine will.

This secret of taking dominion when praying is crucial in the moving of mountains. Christ did not say that we should pray for God to come and move the mountain. He said, "If *you* say to this mountain, 'Be removed and be cast into the sea,' it will be done" (Matt. 21:21).

When Moses had reached the Red Sea, he found that he was closed in by mountains on both sides and by the sea in front of him. Behind him was the pursuing Egyptian army. The situation was desperate. Although God had promised He would fight for the children of Israel, with the bloodthirsty host of Pharaoh hot on their trail and the terrified Israelites losing faith in his leadership, Moses was no doubt uneasy.

WHEN GOD REBUKED MOSES FOR PRAYING

Moses prayed, pleading with God to come to the rescue. In order to escape, the mountains that hemmed them in must be moved or else the Red Sea must be opened. God's answer was a strange one. He rebuked Moses for praying! There are times when we should pray, but this was not one of those times. This was the time for action! Now was the time to speak to the sea to divide!

And the LORD said to Moses, "Why do you cry to Me?
Tell the children of Israel to go forward. But lift up your
rod, and stretch out your hand over the sea and divide it.
And the children of Israel shall go on dry ground through
the midst of the sea" (Ex. 14:15,16).

The reason many prayers are not answered quickly or at all is that believers are not doing their full part. They do not follow up their prayers by using the authority God has given them. Moses had prayed. But now it was time for action. Recognizing his mistake, he stretched out his rod out over the sea — and the water divided!

Acting on our faith after we have prayed is one of the most plainly taught lessons of the Bible.

All through the Scriptures, people of God put their faith into action after they prayed. Joshua spoke to the sun and moon in the valley of Aijalon, and they stood still. Elijah spoke and there was no rain for three years. He spoke again, and the widow's oil and flour lasted during the whole time of famine. He spoke yet again, and there was sound of abundance of rain.

The New Testament, too, is full of examples of action. Jesus was certainly a man of prayer. But it was when He spoke that the water was turned into wine. It was when He spoke that the leper was healed. It was at His word that the wind became still and the sea calm. It was at His command that demons were forced to come out. It was when He whispered that the blind saw and the deaf heard. Jesus spoke words of judgment to the barren fig tree and it dried up from the roots. He commanded and Lazarus, who had been dead four days, came out of the tomb.

The disciples watched Jesus as He worked and they, too, learned the secret of command. They, too, began to do the works He did. Jesus gave them the use of His name, and when they spoke the word, miracles took place.

At the Beautiful Gate, Peter said to the lame man, "Silver and gold I do not have, but what I do have I give you: In the name of Jesus Christ of Nazareth, rise up and walk" (Acts 3:6). And this man who had not walked since he was born, leaped up and walked.

Paul spoke to the false prophet who tried to resist his preaching of the Gospel, and a dark mist fell on him (Acts 13:9-11). He spoke to the demon in the fortune-telling girl, and that very hour the evil spirit left her (Acts 16:18).

Is it dangerous for us to have such power? Only if we use it for selfish purposes. Only if we fail to be led by the Spirit. It is possible for men and women to do so, and we must be careful to exercise this God-given power properly. Moses lifted his rod and struck a rock twice, commanding water to come out (Num. 20:10,11). The water came, but since the act was done in anger rather than in the Spirit of God, Moses was not permitted to lead the children of Israel into the Promised Land (Num. 20:12).

Jesus said, "If you say to this mountain, 'Be removed and be cast into the sea,' it will be done" (Matt. 21:21). We must speak to the mountain, not wait for God to speak to it. We must use the authority God has given us. If we will speak, God will speak. If we will act, God will act. He has given us His name and His authority.

THE SNOWSTORM IN THE SIERRAS

Years ago, as a young evangelist, I was invited to preach in a village high up in the Sierra mountains of California. After praying about the matter, I scheduled a series of services for a certain date.

When the time came to leave for the meetings, a heavy rain was falling in the valley. A long-time resident informed me that rain this time of year meant snow in the mountains, and in all probability, it had been snowing up there for many hours. I was also told that at that time of year, snow often continued to fall for many days, shutting down all travel to the mountain villages on the other side of the pass. This information disturbed me, but I didn't feel right in waiting several days until the storm was over, because I would miss my appointment.

Taking the precaution to purchase rope chains, I took off. As I had been warned, half way up the mountain, the rain turned to snow. However, it seemed there was nothing to do but to go on. The snow gradually got deeper, and after awhile I installed the rope chains. This gave me better traction, but the depth of the snow constantly increased. At one of the villages on the ascent, I was informed it had been snowing on the summit for 72 hours and the snow there was probably over a foot deep. Since there was no indication of a letup, there was slim chance of getting through for several days. However, I continued on. I had promised to begin the services on the following night, and I decided to go as far as I could.

But I could not get much further right then. The snow became so deep the car finally stalled. Unless the storm ceased, I was in real trouble. Now I had to have a miracle. The blizzard must stop, if the snow plow was to come through in the morning. Ordinarily, I would not have had faith to pray for a snow storm to stop. But up on the high Sierras, cut off from the world, it was different. The Spirit of God was there.

Wrapping some blankets around me, I began to pray. Humanly speaking, I was alone; but I knew God was with me in the car. I told Him I was making this journey for His glory; that I had an appointment the following day to preach His Gospel and I must get through. Although snow had fallen for many hours, and in the natural there was every indication that it would continue, I needed the storm to stop. As I prayed, a boldness came over me. I felt an authority to command the storm to stop. How long I prayed I don't know. But suddenly I knew the answer had come!

I opened my eyes and I looked at the sky that a few moments before was covered with heavy clouds. Now the stars were shining brightly and there was only a slight trace of a cloud remaining. I went to sleep and was awakened with sunlight streaming through the car windows. An hour or two later, the snow plow came through. That night, I began services in the little chapel as I had promised.

Man was made in the image of God and given dominion over the earth. Christ restored that dominion by giving us His power and His authority. There is a time to pray, and there is a time to act. There is a time to take authority. There is a time when a believer, like Moses, must rise from prayer, lift up his or her rod and speak to the sea to divide. Jesus said that if we speak in faith, it shall be done.

CHAPTER XIX

The Secret of Prayer Without Ceasing

Then He spoke a parable to them, that men always ought
to pray and not lose heart (Lk. 18:1).

When Jesus answered the disciples' request to teach them how
to pray, He gave a parable to bring home His final important point
concerning the art of successful prayer. To receive the answer, we
must be steadfast and determined. We must not allow
discouragement to cause us to faint.

Jesus told about a man whose friend arrived at midnight from a
long journey — hungry and tired. Unfortunately, the man had
nothing to give him. So, he went to another friend and asked to
borrow three loaves of bread. The friend, annoyed at being disturbed
at that hour of the night, said his children were asleep, and he did
not want to wake up his entire household. Rather gruffly, he told the
man to stop bothering him and go back home. But the man was
persistent, and continued knocking on the door. Jesus then said, "I
say to you, though he will not rise and give to him because he is his
friend, yet because of his persistence he will rise and give him as
many as he needs" (Lk. 11:8).

Here is the final lesson on prayer. It sums up all other lessons.
We must be determined to get the answer. The parable on persistence
assumes there will be difficulties — times when it seems that our

prayer will not be answered. We are not to be discouraged, but persevere; we must never give up. In the end, the answer will come! Jesus concluded His lesson with these words:

> And I say to you, ask, and it will be given to you; seek, and you will find; knock, and it will be opened to you. For everyone who asks receives, and he who seeks finds, and to him who knocks it will be opened (Lk. 11:9,10).

PARABLE OF THE UNJUST JUDGE

The Lord repeated His admonition to persevere in prayer — "that men always ought to pray and not lose heart" (Lk. 18:1) — by giving them another parable. In a certain city was a judge who did not fear God nor respect men. A widow came to him asking for justice. For a while he paid no attention to her. But because she kept coming, he finally gave in. "Then the Lord said, 'And shall God not avenge His own elect who cry out day and night to Him, though He bears long with them? I tell you that He will avenge them speedily. Nevertheless, when the Son of Man comes, will He really find faith on the earth?'" (Lk. 18:6-8).

So Christ encouraged His disciples to be constant in prayer, to pray without ceasing, to always pray and not to faint. God will take care of His part. The only issue in doubt is whether we will do our part. Our faith will not fail if we keep our eyes upon the promise and place God's word above all else.

When Jacob's brother Esau came with 400 men of war, Jacob was in the greatest crisis of his life. But he said to the angel, "I will not let You go unless You bless me!" (Gen. 32:26). And the angel blessed him.

When because of the Israelites' sin, the Lord refused to go with them into Canaan, Moses said, "If Your Presence does not go with us, do not bring us up from here" (Ex. 33:15). God granted his request and said, "My Presence will go with you, and I will give you rest" (Ex. 33:14).

Elijah prayed seven times that the Lord would send rain to Israel and bring an end to the famine. The rain came.

Daniel interceded for 21 days, not knowing the "prince of Persia" was hindering the answer to his prayer. He held on until the answer came.

We could go on naming the men and women in God's hall of faith. They refused to be defeated or accept failure; they held on until the answer came. Jesus said, "Men always ought to pray and not lose heart" (Lk. 18:1). If there are hindrances, things standing in the way or conditions to be met, the important thing is to stand steady, never giving any ground to the enemy. The answer will come in due time.

WHEN THE EISENHOWER FAMILY PRAYED WITHOUT CEASING

Proof that prevailing prayer overcomes all obstacles was demonstrated by the famous Eisenhower family. Had that family not known how to pray, the life of Dwight Eisenhower, who was to become president of the United States, could have been lost, and world history would have been much different. This story appeared in the *Reader's Digest,* and its authenticity is unquestioned.

As a young boy, Dwight fell while running home from school and injured his leg. At first he didn't notice any pain, but by evening the knee started to ache. He said his prayers and went to bed.

The leg was quite painful by morning. But Dwight did his chores because everybody in his family had to work. Two mornings later his leg was so bad that he couldn't get as far as the barn. By noon he was forced to go to bed. His mother was alarmed. She bathed the infection, applied poultices and called the doctor.

Dr. Conklin examined the leg and said that it was not likely it could be saved. When the boy heard this, he cried out, "Don't take off my leg. I would rather die!" But the doctor replied, "The longer we wait, the more we will have to take off." When the doctor went out of the room, Dwight called his brother into the room and said,

"If I go out of my head, don't let them take off my leg." The brother accepted the responsibility.

The mother and father were not convinced that amputation was necessary, and with the son's stand, they decided not to yield to the doctor's advice. But the fever mounted, and the discoloration was hourly climbing higher on Dwight's limb, just as the doctor said it would.

The parents were in a dilemma. The doctor angrily declared they were responsible for the boy's life. Suddenly, they all thought of the same thing. Had they forgotten their faith in God, and that their minister had always believed in healing through faith? In this desperate hour, they all took turns praying at the bedside. Some would rise and go about their work, but at least one would continue in prayer. All the four brothers joined in this prayer vigil that was kept around the clock.

When the doctor returned, his experienced eye saw a change. The discoloration was vanishing, and the swelling going down. Dwight's life was saved! Their faith in the God of miracles was not in vain.

The family of Dwight Eisenhower, later to become the President of the United States, prayed until they received the answer. God grant that all the people of America learn to pray with such persistence.

DON'T FAINT — YOUR PRAYER WILL BE ANSWERED

Jesus told us to pray and not faint. "For everyone who asks receives, and he who seeks finds, and to him who knocks it will be opened" (Lk. 11:10).

God promised Abraham He would give him the land of Canaan — the land stretching all the way from the Euphrates River to the Great Sea. Yet when Abraham's wife, Sarah, died, he was obliged to pay 400 pieces of silver for a plot of ground large enough for a burial place. Four centuries later, through a series of great miracles, God took the seed of Abraham out of Egypt and gave them the land He had promised.

Jacob vowed to the Lord that if He would be with him and give him clothing and bread to eat, he would serve Him all the days of his life. But a time of severe testing came to the patriarch. After years of prosperity, everything seemed to go wrong. His favorite son, Joseph, disappeared and for many years he supposed him dead. A famine came, and when the family of Jacob tried to obtain food in Egypt, the ruler of that country treated Jacob's sons roughly and put one of them in prison. It seemed that God had forgotten Jacob, and that he and all his family would soon perish. But God had not forgotten Jacob's prayer. All the time He was working things out for good. Joseph, who had been sold into Egypt by his brothers, had risen to great power and become ruler of Egypt. Under the most touching circumstances, Joseph made himself known to his brothers. It turned out that the very things that Jacob thought could only bring him evil, God used to bless him and his family and bring a mighty deliverance.

Mary and Martha asked Jesus to come and heal their brother Lazarus. But Lazarus died and was buried. Had Jesus failed? The Lord met the sisters in their great sorrow and said, "Did I not say to you that if you would believe you would see the glory of God?" (Jn. 11:40). To the unspeakable joy of the sisters, their brother Lazarus was brought to life and the little family was reunited. Their prayer had been answered!

Stephen, the first martyr, prayed for God to forgive the men who were stoning him. Was his prayer answered? Saul of Tarsus, the ring leader and chief persecutor of the Christians, stood holding the coats of those who did the stoning, looking on with grim satisfaction. But Saul, later called Paul, became Christianity's most famous convert, and its greatest champion. Was not Stephen's prayer answered, even beyond what he had hoped?

For nineteen hundred years the Church has been praying, "Your kingdom come. Your will be done on earth as it is in heaven" (Matt. 6:10). Some say that Jesus will never return and His Kingdom will never come. But over the centuries, God has one-by-one gathered the prayers of His saints. It is almost time for the great angel to take those prayers and offer them in the censer before the throne of God. Christ's kingdom will come! His will shall be done on earth as it is in heaven! Amen.

SPECIAL NOTE: A free gift subscription to CHRIST FOR THE NATIONS magazine is available to those who write to Christ For The Nations, P.O. Box 769000, Dallas, TX 75376-9000. This magazine contains special feature stories of men of faith and includes prophetic articles on the latest world developments. Why not include the names of your friends? (Due to high mailing rates, this applies only to Canada and the U.S.)